Nursing
Calculations

J. D. Gatford

Mathematics Teacher
Langwarrin Secondary
College, Victoria

Churchill Livingstone

MELBOURNE EDINBURGH LONDON AND NEW YORK 1987

CHURCHILL LIVINGSTONE
Medical Division of Longman Group UK Limited

Distributed in the Australia by Longman Cheshire Pty Limited,
Longman House, Kings Gardens, 95 Coventry Street, South
Melbourne 3205, and by associated companies, branches and
representatives throughout the world.

First edition 1982
Second edition 1987
 Reprinted 1988

ISBN 0-443-03533-4

British Library Cataloguing in Publication Data
Gatford, J.D.
  Nursing calculations. – 2nd ed.
  1. Nursing — Mathematics — Problems, exercises,
  etc. 2. Arithmetic — Problems, exercises, etc.
  1. Title.
  513'.024613   RT68

Library of Congress Cataloging in Publication Data
Gatford, J.D.
  Nursing calculations.
  1. Pharmaceutical arithmetic. 2. Nursing — Mathematics.
  I. Title. [DNLM: 1. Drugs — administration & dosage — nurses'
  instruction.
  2. Mathematics — nurses' instruction. QV 16 G255n]
  RS57.G38   1986   513'.024613   86–17145

Produced by Longman Singapore Publishers (Pte) Ltd.
Printed in Singapore.

Nursing
Calculations

The author and his family dedicate this second edition of *Nursing Calculations* to the memory of our dear friend Sandy who died suddenly, at the age of 17, of a rare illness known as Goodpasture's syndrome.

Preface to the Second Edition

The author would like to thank those nurse educators who offered constructive criticism of the first edition.

This second edition has an additional exercise on drip rates involving simple changes in the rate. Also, two comprehensive summary exercises have been included, after the topic chapters. These exercises can be used to revise all of the nursing topics.

Further suggestions and comments would be greatly appreciated.

Melbourne 1987   J.D.G.

Acknowledgements

The author and publishers would like to thank many students and nurses in hospitals around Australia for providing advice and criticism during the preparation of this book. Special thanks are extended to staff at Royal Children's Hospital, Melbourne; Prince Henry's Hospital, Melbourne; Alfred Hospital, Melbourne; and Bethesda Hospital, Melbourne.

The author wishes also to thank: his friends, Cec Pitman and Marj Dannatt, for their assistance in the checking of answers; and his wife, Elaine, for related secretarial work, and especially for her patience.

Preface to the First Edition

This book was written at the request of nurse educators and with considerable help from them. It deals with elements of the arithmetic of nursing, especially the arithmetic of basic pharmacology.

The book begins with a diagnostic test which is carefully related to a set of review exercises in basic arithmetic. Answers to the test are supplied at the back of the book, and are keyed to the corresponding review exercises.

Students should work through those exercises which correspond to errors in the diagnostic test. The other exercises may also, of course, be worked through to improve speed and accuracy.

Throughout the other chapters of the book there are adequate, well graded exercise and problems. Each chapter includes several worked examples. Answers are given to all questions.

Suggestions and comments from nurse educators and students on the scope and content of this book would be welcomed. The hope is that its relevance to nursing needs will be maintained in subsequent editions.

Melbourne 1982   J.D.G.

Contents

1. A review of basic calculations

The chapter begins with a diagnostic test. This is designed to pinpoint those areas of your arithmetic which need revising before you commence nursing calculations.

Attempt all questions.

Answers are supplied at the back of the book, and direct you to particular exercises, according to the *errors* in your test answers.

For example, if you make an error in answering either question 1 or question 2, then you will be asked to do Exercise 1A. Or, if your answer to question 3 or 4 is wrong, you should do Exercise 1B.

Work carefully and neatly.

Remember that this test is designed to *help* you.

Diagnostic test

1. Multiply
   (a) 83×10 (b) 83×100 (c) 83×1000

2. Multiply
   (a) $0 \cdot 0258 \times 10$ (b) $0 \cdot 0258 \times 100$
   (c) $0 \cdot 0258 \times 1000$

3. Divide. Write answers as decimals.
   (a) $3 \cdot 78 \div 10$ (b) $3 \cdot 78 \div 100$ (c) $3 \cdot 78 \div 1000$

4. Divide. Write answers as decimals.
   (a) $\dfrac{569}{10}$ (b) $\dfrac{569}{100}$ (c) $\dfrac{569}{1000}$

5. Complete
   (a) 1 gram   = ... milligrams
   (b) 1 milligram = ... micrograms
   (c) 1 litre   = ... millilitres

Write answers to (6), (7) and (8) in decimal form:

6. (a) Change $0 \cdot 78$ grams to milligrams
   (b) Change 34 milligrams to grams

7. (a) Change 0·086 mg to micrograms
   (b) Change 294 micrograms to mg

8. (a) Change 2·4 litres to millilitres
   (b) Change 965 millilitres to litres

9. Evaluate (multiply)
   (a) 9×3 (b) $0·9 \times 3$
   (c) $0·9 \times 0·3$ (d) $0·09 \times 0·03$

10. Evaluate (multiply)
    (a) 78×6 (b) $7·8 \times 0·6$
    (c) $0·78 \times 6$ (d) $7·8 \times 0·06$

11. Calculate the volume of distilled water which must be added to 175 ml of stock solution to make 850 ml of diluted solution.

12. Calculate the volume of distilled water which must be added to 350 ml of stock solution to make $2\frac{1}{2}$ litres of diluted solution.

13. Which of the numbers 2, 3, 5, 6, 7, 9, 11 are FACTORS of 126?

14. Simplify ('cancel down')

    (a) $\dfrac{16}{24}$ (b) $\dfrac{56}{72}$

15. Simplify

(a) $\dfrac{45}{600}$ (b) $\dfrac{175}{400}$

16. Simplify

(a) $\dfrac{40}{50}$ (b) $\dfrac{60}{90}$ (c) $\dfrac{90}{150}$

17. Simplify

(a) $\dfrac{350}{500}$ (b) $\dfrac{1200}{1500}$ (c) $\dfrac{1600}{4000}$

18. Write correct to one decimal place

(a) 0·87   (b) 0·63   (c) 0·49

19. Change to decimals correct to *one* decimal place

(a) $\dfrac{1}{6}$ (b) $\dfrac{3}{7}$ (c) $\dfrac{7}{9}$

20. Change to exact decimal equivalents

(a) $\dfrac{5}{8}$ (b) $\dfrac{9}{20}$ (c) $\dfrac{17}{25}$ (d) $\dfrac{31}{40}$

21. Change to decimals correct to *two* decimal places

(a) $\dfrac{5}{7}$ (b) $\dfrac{7}{9}$

22. Change to decimals correct to *three* decimal places

    (a) $\dfrac{7}{30}$ (b) $\dfrac{59}{70}$

23. Change to a percentage

    (a) $\dfrac{3}{4}$ (b) $\dfrac{13}{20}$ (c) $\dfrac{8}{25}$

24. Change to a percentage

    (a) $\dfrac{1}{3}$ (b) $\dfrac{5}{8}$ (c) $\dfrac{5}{9}$

25. Change these ratios to the form 1 in x
    (a) 1:4   (b) 1:20

26. Change these ratios to the form 1:y
    (a) 1 in 4   (b) 1 in 30

27. How much stock solution is present in 600 ml of solution if the dilution ratio is 1 in 3?

28. How much stock solution is present in 400 ml of solution if the dilution ratio is 1:4?

29. Change each ratio to a percentage
    (a) 1 in 5   (b) 1 in 50
    (c) 1 in 500   (d) 1 in 5000

30. Change to a vulgar fraction and simplify where possible

    (a) 0·3   (b) 0·6   (c) 0·8

31. Change to a vulgar fraction and simplify where possible

    (a) 0.55   (b) 0·72   (c) 0·68   (d) 0·09

32. Change to a vulgar fraction and simplify where possible

    (a) 6%   (b) 43%   (c) 75%

33. Change to a vulgar fraction and simplify if possible

    (a) 0·7%   (b) 0·03%   (c) 0·05%

34. Change to a vulgar fraction and simplify if possible

    (a) $\frac{1}{2}$%   (b) $5\frac{1}{2}$%   (c) $17\frac{1}{2}$%

35. Multiply. Simplify where possible

    (a) $\frac{2}{3} \times \frac{5}{6}$ (b) $\frac{5}{8} \times \frac{12}{7}$ (c) $\frac{9}{10} \times \frac{4}{9}$

36. Divide. Simplify where possible

    (a) $\frac{1}{3} \div \frac{1}{5}$ (b) $\frac{3}{7} \div \frac{3}{5}$ (c) $\frac{5}{8} \div \frac{7}{10}$

37. Refer to the tables on page 43. Change these heights to centimetres (to nearest cm)

    (a) 3′ 10″   (b) 4′ 5″   (c) 5′ 8″

38. Refer to the tables on pages 44 and 45. Change these weights to kilograms (to nearest kg)

(a)   7 st 6 lb

(b)   10 st 10 lb

(c)   13 st 8 lb

Multiplication by 10, 100 and 1000

EXAMPLES

(i) 0·36 × 10 (ii) 0·36 × 100 (iii) 0·36 × 1000

Long method

(i)	0·36	(ii)	0·36	(iii)	0·36
	× 10		× 100		× 1000
	3·60		36·00		360·00

Short method

(i) 0·36 × 10   = 3·6   = 3·6

(ii) 0·36 × 100   = 36·   = 36

(iii) 0·36 × 1000 = 360· = 360

NOTES (a) Use zeros to make up places, where necessary.

(b) If the answer is a whole number, the decimal point may be omitted.

SUMMARY OF SHORT METHOD

To MULTIPLY by	Move the decimal point
10	1 place right
100	2 places right
1000	3 places right

EXERCISE 1A   Multiply.

(1) 0·68 × 10
0·68 × 100
0·68 × 1000

(2) 0·975 × 10
0·975 × 100
0·975 × 1000

(3) 3·7 × 10
3·7 × 100
3·7 × 1000

(4) 5·62 × 10
5·62 × 100
5·62 × 1000

(5) 77 × 10
77 × 100
77 × 1000

(6) 825 × 10
825 × 100
825 × 1000

(7) 0·2 × 10
0·2 × 100
0·2 × 1000

(8) 0·046 × 10
0·046 × 100
0·046 × 1000

(9) 0·0147 × 10
0·0147 × 100
0·0147 × 1000

(10) 0·006 × 10
0·006 × 100
0·006 × 1000

(11) 3·76 × 10
3·76 × 100
3·76 × 1000

(12) 0·639 × 10
0·639 × 100
0·639 × 1000

(13) 0·075 × 10
0·075 × 100
0·075 × 1000

(14) 0·08 × 10
0·08 × 100
0·08 × 1000

(15) 0·003 × 10
0·003 × 100
0·003 × 1000

(16) 0·0505 × 10
0·0505 × 100
0·0505 × 1000

Division by 10, 100 and 1000

EXAMPLE A

    Short method

  (i) **37·8 ÷ 10**   (i) $37·8 ÷ 10 = 3\overset{\frown}{·}78$

  (ii) **37·8 ÷ 100**   (ii) $37·8 ÷ 100 = 0\overset{\frown}{·}378$

 (iii) **37·8 ÷ 1000** (iii) $37·8 ÷ 1000 = 0\overset{\frown}{·}0378$

NOTES **(a) Use zeros to make up places, where necessary.**

           (b) Write a zero before the decimal point [for numbers less than one].

EXAMPLE B
A division may be written as a fraction.

Evaluate   **(i)** $\dfrac{\mathbf{0·984}}{\mathbf{10}}$ (i) $\dfrac{0·984}{10} = 0·0984$

         (ii) $\dfrac{\mathbf{0·984}}{\mathbf{100}}$ (ii) $\dfrac{0·984}{100} = 0·00984$

        (iii) $\dfrac{\mathbf{0·984}}{\mathbf{1000}}$ (iii) $\dfrac{0·984}{1000} = 0·000984$

SUMMARY OF SHORT METHOD

To DIVIDE by	Move the decimal point
10	1 place left
100	2 places left
1000	3 places left

EXERCISE 1B   Divide. Write answers as decimals.

(1) $98\cdot4 \div 10$
         $98\cdot4 \div 100$
         $98\cdot4 \div 1000$

(2) $5\cdot91 \div 10$
         $5\cdot91 \div 100$
         $5\cdot91 \div 1000$

(3) $2\cdot6 \div 10$
         $2\cdot6 \div 100$
         $2\cdot6 \div 1000$

(4) $307 \div 10$
         $307 \div 100$
         $307 \div 1000$

(5) $82 \div 10$
         $82 \div 100$
         $82 \div 1000$

(6) $7 \div 10$
         $7 \div 100$
         $7 \div 1000$

(7) $3 \div 10$
         $3 \div 100$
         $3 \div 1000$

(8) $7\cdot5 \div 10$
         $7\cdot5 \div 100$
         $7\cdot5 \div 1000$

(9) $\dfrac{68}{10}$

         $\dfrac{68}{100}$

         $\dfrac{68}{1000}$

(10) $\dfrac{2\cdot29}{10}$

         $\dfrac{2\cdot29}{100}$

         $\dfrac{2\cdot29}{1000}$

(11) $\dfrac{51\cdot4}{10}$

         $\dfrac{51\cdot4}{100}$

         $\dfrac{51\cdot4}{1000}$

(12) $\dfrac{916}{10}$

         $\dfrac{916}{100}$

         $\dfrac{916}{1000}$

(13) $\dfrac{67\cdot2}{10}$

         $\dfrac{67\cdot2}{100}$

         $\dfrac{67\cdot2}{1000}$

(14) $\dfrac{387}{10}$

         $\dfrac{387}{100}$

         $\dfrac{387}{1000}$

(15) $\dfrac{8\cdot94}{10}$

         $\dfrac{8\cdot94}{100}$

         $\dfrac{8\cdot94}{1000}$

(16) $\dfrac{0\cdot707}{10}$

         $\dfrac{0\cdot707}{100}$

         $\dfrac{0\cdot707}{1000}$

Converting metric units

MEMORISE

> **1 gram (g) = 1000 milligrams (mg)**
> **1 milligram (mg) = 1000 micrograms (μg)**
> **1 litre (l) = 1000 millilitres (ml)**

EXAMPLE A   Change 0·67 grams to mg

$$0·67\,g = 0·67 \times 1000\,mg$$
$$= 670\,mg$$

EXAMPLE B   Change 23 mg to grams

$$23\,mg = 23 \div 1000\,g$$
$$= 0·023\,g$$

EXAMPLE C   Change 0·075 mg to micrograms

$$0·075\,mg = 0·075 \times 1000\,micrograms$$
$$= 75\,micrograms$$

It is better to write the word micrograms than use the symbol μg

EXAMPLE D   Change 185 micrograms to mg

$$185\,micrograms = 185 \div 1000\,mg$$
$$= 0·185\,mg$$

EXAMPLE E   Change 1·3 litres to ml

$$1·3\,litres = 1·3 \times 1000\,ml$$
$$= 1300\,ml$$

EXAMPLE F   Change 850 ml to litres

$$850\,ml = 850 \div 1000\,litres$$
$$= 0·85\,litres$$

EXERCISE 1C   Write all answers in decimal form.

Change to milligrams

(1) 4 g   **(3)** 0·69 g   **(5)** 0·035 g   **(7)** 0·655 g

(2) 8·7 g   **(4)** 0·02 g   **(6)** 0·006 g   **(8)** 4·28 g

Change to grams

(9) 6000 mg   **(11)** 865 mg   **(13)** 70 mg   **(15)** 5 mg

(10) 7250 mg   **(12)** 95 mg   **(14)** 2 mg   **(16)** 125 mg

Change to micrograms

(17) 0·195 mg   **(20)** 0·075 mg   **(23)** 0·625 mg

(18) 0·6 mg   **(21)** 0·08 mg   **(24)** 0·098 mg

(19) 0·75 mg   **(22)** 0·001 mg

Change to milligrams

(25) 825 micrograms   **(29)** 10 micrograms

(26) 750 micrograms   **(30)** 5 micrograms

(27) 65 micrograms   **(31)** 200 micrograms

(28) 95 micrograms   **(32)** 30 micrograms

Change to millilitres

(33) 2 litres   **(36)** 4½ litres   **(39)** 0·8 litres

(34) 30 litres   **(37)** 1·6 litres   **(40)** 0·75 litres

(35) 1½ litres   **(38)** 2·24 litres

Change to litres

(41) 4000 ml   **(43)** 625 ml   **(45)** 95 ml   **(47)** 5 ml

(42) 10 000 ml   **(44)** 350 ml   **(46)** 60 ml   **(48)** 2 ml

Multiplication of decimals

Note: d.p. is used in the examples to stand for 'decimal places'.

EXAMPLE A Evaluate
(a) 8×4
(b) 0.8×4
(c) 0.8×0.4
(d) 0.08×0.04

EXAMPLE B Evaluate
(a) 67×4
(b) 6.7×0.4
(c) 0.67×4
(d) 6.7×0.04

(a) $8 \times 4 = 32$

(b) $0.8 \times 4 = 3.2$
1 d.p. + 0 d.p. $\Rightarrow$ 1 d.p.

(c) $0.8 \times 0.4 = 0.32$
1 d.p. + 1 d.p. $\Rightarrow$ 2 d.p.

(d) $0.08 \times 0.04 = 0.0032$
2 d.p. + 2 d.p. $\Rightarrow$ 4 d.p.

(a) $67 \times 4 = 268$

(b) $6.7 \times 0.4 = 2.68$
1 d.p. + 1 d.p. $\Rightarrow$ 2 d.p.

(c) $0.67 \times 4 = 2.68$
2 d.p. + 0 d.p. $\Rightarrow$ 2 d.p.

(d) $6.7 \times 0.04 = 0.268$
1 d.p. + 2 d.p. $\Rightarrow$ 3 d.p.

EXAMPLE C Evaluate
(a) 16×12
(b) 1.6×1.2
(c) 0.16×0.12
(d) 0.016×1.2

(a) $16 \times 12 = 192$
(b) $1.6 \times 1.2 = 1.92$
(c) $0.16 \times 0.12 = 0.0192$
(d) $0.016 \times 1.2 = 0.0192$

EXERCISE 1D   Evaluate.

1. 9×5
$0 \cdot 9 \times 5$
$0 \cdot 9 \times 0 \cdot 5$
$9 \times 0 \cdot 05$

6. 17×6
$1 \cdot 7 \times 6$
$0 \cdot 17 \times 6$
$0 \cdot 17 \times 0 \cdot 6$

11. 37×9
$3 \cdot 7 \times 9$
$3 \cdot 7 \times 0 \cdot 09$
$0 \cdot 37 \times 0 \cdot 09$

2. 2×7
$0 \cdot 2 \times 0 \cdot 7$
$0 \cdot 2 \times 0 \cdot 07$
$0 \cdot 02 \times 0 \cdot 07$

7. 19×8
$19 \times 0 \cdot 8$
$0 \cdot 19 \times 0 \cdot 8$
$1 \cdot 9 \times 0 \cdot 08$

12. 41×7
$0 \cdot 41 \times 0 \cdot 7$
$0 \cdot 41 \times 0 \cdot 07$
$4 \cdot 1 \times 0 \cdot 7$

3. 3×4
$3 \times 0 \cdot 04$
$0 \cdot 3 \times 0 \cdot 4$
$0 \cdot 03 \times 0 \cdot 04$

8. 23×2
$2 \cdot 3 \times 0 \cdot 2$
$2 \cdot 3 \times 0 \cdot 02$
$2 \cdot 3 \times 0 \cdot 002$

13. 48×4
$0 \cdot 48 \times 0 \cdot 04$
$48 \times 0 \cdot 004$
$0 \cdot 048 \times 0 \cdot 4$

4. 6×6
$0 \cdot 6 \times 0 \cdot 6$
$0 \cdot 06 \times 0 \cdot 06$
$0 \cdot 6 \times 0 \cdot 006$

9. 29×5
$0 \cdot 29 \times 5$
$2 \cdot 9 \times 0 \cdot 5$
$29 \times 0 \cdot 05$

14. 56×11
$5 \cdot 6 \times 1 \cdot 1$
$0 \cdot 56 \times 0 \cdot 11$
$56 \times 0 \cdot 011$

5. 7×8
$0 \cdot 7 \times 8$
$0 \cdot 7 \times 0 \cdot 8$
$0 \cdot 07 \times 0 \cdot 08$

10. 31×3
$3 \cdot 1 \times 0 \cdot 3$
$0 \cdot 31 \times 0 \cdot 03$
$31 \times 0 \cdot 003$

15. 64×12
$6 \cdot 4 \times 0 \cdot 12$
$0 \cdot 64 \times 0 \cdot 12$
$0 \cdot 064 \times 1 \cdot 2$

Diluting solutions

Stock solutions must often be diluted to obtain the strength required for a patient's treatment.

Dilution is usually done by mixing stock solution with distilled water.

EXAMPLE

Calculate the volume of distilled water which must be added to 375 ml of stock solution to make 3 litres of diluted solution.

3 litres = 3000 ml

$$\begin{array}{r} 3000 \\ 375 \\ \hline \end{array} -$$

2625 ml of distilled water

EXERCISE 1E Calculate the amount of distilled water which must be added to the stock solution to make up the total volume required.

	Total volume required	Volume of stock solution		Total volume required	Volume of stock solution
1	600 ml	100 ml	**16**	2 litres	350 ml
2	600 ml	150 ml	**17**	2 litres	425 ml
3	600 ml	75 ml	**18**	2 litres	215 ml
4	750 ml	250 ml	**19**	$1\frac{1}{2}$ litres	150 ml
5	750 ml	125 ml	**20**	$1\frac{1}{2}$ litres	175 ml
6	750 ml	275 ml	**21**	$1\frac{1}{2}$ litres	235 ml
7	1000 ml	200 ml	**22**	$3\frac{1}{2}$ litres	800 ml
8	1000 ml	150 ml	**23**	$3\frac{1}{2}$ litres	650 ml
9	1000 ml	85 ml	**24**	$3\frac{1}{2}$ litres	195 ml
10	1200 ml	250 ml	**25**	3·2 litres	350 ml
11	1200 ml	165 ml	**26**	3·2 litres	475 ml
12	1200 ml	375 ml	**27**	3·2 litres	235 ml
13	1 litre	180 ml	**28**	4·5 litres	150 ml
14	1 litre	225 ml	**29**	4·5 litres	510 ml
15	1 litre	45 ml	**30**	4·5 litres	625 ml

Factors

Many calculations involve the simplifying (or 'cancelling down') of fractions.

This requires a knowledge of FACTORS. When a number is divided by one of its factors, the answer is a whole number (i.e. there is no remainder).

EXAMPLE
   Which of the numbers 2, 3, 5, 7, 11 are factors of 154?

$$2\overline{)154} \qquad 3\overline{)154} \qquad 5\overline{)154} \qquad 7\overline{)154} \qquad 11\overline{)154}$$
$$\quad 77 \qquad\quad 51\tfrac{1}{3} \qquad\quad 30\tfrac{4}{5} \qquad\quad 22 \qquad\qquad 14$$

∴ 2, 7 and 11 are factors of 154.

NOTES (a) These are not the ONLY factors of 154.
   (b) The numbers can, of course, be checked mentally!

EXERCISE IF Which of the numbers in Column B are factors of the number (opposite) in Column A?

	A	B
1	20	2, 3, 4, 5, 7, 8
2	36	3, 4, 5, 10, 12, 16
3	45	3, 5, 7, 11, 12, 15
4	56	2, 5, 8, 11, 14, 16
5	60	3, 4, 8, 12, 15, 20
6	72	3, 4, 6, 12, 15, 18
7	75	3, 5, 7, 11, 15, 25
8	85	3, 5, 9, 11, 15, 17
9	96	3, 8, 12, 14, 16, 24
10	100	3, 5, 8, 20, 25, 40
11	108	4, 7, 9, 12, 16, 18
12	120	3, 5, 9, 12, 15, 16
13	135	3, 5, 7, 9, 11, 15
14	144	4, 8, 12, 16, 18, 24
15	150	4, 5, 9, 12, 15, 25
16	165	3, 5, 7, 9, 11, 15
17	175	3, 5, 7, 9, 11, 15
18	180	4, 8, 12, 15, 16, 25
19	192	4, 6, 8, 12, 15, 16
20	210	4, 6, 9, 12, 14, 15

Simplifying fractions 1

To simplify (or 'cancel down') a fraction, divide the numerator *and* the denominator by the *same* number. This number is called a COMMON FACTOR.

EXAMPLE A   Simplify $\frac{36}{48}$

$\frac{36}{48} = \frac{3}{4}$ $\begin{bmatrix} \text{After dividing numerator and} \\ \text{denominator by 12} \end{bmatrix}$

Or this may be done in two or more steps:

$\frac{36}{48} = \frac{18}{24}$ $\begin{bmatrix} \text{Dividing numerator and} \\ \text{denominator by 2} \end{bmatrix}$

$= \frac{9}{12}$ $\begin{bmatrix} \text{Again dividing numerator and} \\ \text{denominator by 2} \end{bmatrix}$

$= \frac{3}{4}$ $\begin{bmatrix} \text{Dividing numerator and} \\ \text{denominator by 3} \end{bmatrix}$

Note: $2 \times 2 \times 3 = 12$

EXAMPLE B   Simplify $\frac{125}{225}$

$\frac{125}{225} = \frac{25}{45}$ $\begin{bmatrix} \text{Dividing numerator and} \\ \text{denominator by 5} \end{bmatrix}$

$= \frac{5}{9}$ $\begin{bmatrix} \text{Again dividing numerator and} \\ \text{denominator by 5} \end{bmatrix}$

EXERCISE 1G

Part a   Simplify ('cancel down')

(1) $\frac{8}{12}$ **(6)** $\frac{15}{21}$ **(11)** $\frac{28}{32}$ **(16)** $\frac{14}{42}$ **(21)** $\frac{36}{56}$

(2) $\frac{10}{14}$ **(7)** $\frac{20}{24}$ **(12)** $\frac{22}{33}$ **(17)** $\frac{30}{45}$ **(22)** $\frac{48}{60}$

(3) $\frac{6}{16}$ **(8)** $\frac{20}{25}$ **(13)** $\frac{15}{35}$ **(18)** $\frac{42}{48}$ **(23)** $\frac{52}{64}$

(4) $\frac{9}{18}$ **(9)** $\frac{12}{28}$ **(14)** $\frac{32}{36}$ **(19)** $\frac{36}{50}$ **(24)** $\frac{21}{70}$

(5) $\frac{15}{20}$ **(10)** $\frac{9}{30}$ **(15)** $\frac{16}{40}$ **(20)** $\frac{25}{55}$ **(25)** $\frac{32}{72}$

Part b   Simplify ('cancel down')

(1) $\frac{75}{150}$ **(5)** $\frac{125}{250}$ **(9)** $\frac{30}{225}$ **(13)** $\frac{125}{200}$ **(17)** $\frac{175}{225}$

(2) $\frac{75}{200}$ **(6)** $\frac{125}{300}$ **(10)** $\frac{40}{175}$ **(14)** $\frac{375}{500}$ **(18)** $\frac{225}{300}$

(3) $\frac{75}{250}$ **(7)** $\frac{125}{400}$ **(11)** $\frac{45}{150}$ **(15)** $\frac{275}{400}$ **(19)** $\frac{425}{600}$

(4) $\frac{75}{300}$ **(8)** $\frac{125}{500}$ **(12)** $\frac{60}{375}$ **(16)** $\frac{100}{225}$ **(20)** $\frac{325}{750}$

Simplifying fractions 2

EXAMPLE A Simplify $\dfrac{900}{1500}$

$\dfrac{900}{1500} = \dfrac{9}{15}$ $\left[\begin{array}{l}\text{Dividing numerator and} \\ \text{denominator by 100}\end{array}\right]$

$\qquad\quad = \dfrac{3}{5}$ $\left[\begin{array}{l}\text{Dividing numerator and} \\ \text{denominator by 3}\end{array}\right]$

EXAMPLE B Simplify $\dfrac{1400}{4000}$

$\dfrac{1400}{4000} = \dfrac{14}{40}$ $\left[\begin{array}{l}\text{Dividing numerator and} \\ \text{denominator by 100}\end{array}\right]$

$\qquad\quad = \dfrac{7}{20}$ $\left[\begin{array}{l}\text{Dividing numerator and} \\ \text{denominator by 2}\end{array}\right]$

EXERCISE IH   Divide numerator *and* denominator by 10 or 100 or 1000.

Then simplify further if possible.

(1) $\dfrac{30}{50}$ (10) $\dfrac{120}{160}$ (19) $\dfrac{400}{600}$ (28) $\dfrac{1400}{2500}$

(2) $\dfrac{40}{60}$ (11) $\dfrac{100}{160}$ (20) $\dfrac{450}{600}$ (29) $\dfrac{2000}{2500}$

(3) $\dfrac{60}{80}$ (12) $\dfrac{60}{160}$ (21) $\dfrac{540}{600}$ (30) $\dfrac{1750}{2500}$

(4) $\dfrac{50}{120}$ (13) $\dfrac{200}{300}$ (22) $\dfrac{600}{800}$ (31) $\dfrac{2500}{3000}$

(5) $\dfrac{80}{120}$ (14) $\dfrac{120}{300}$ (23) $\dfrac{750}{800}$ (32) $\dfrac{500}{3000}$

(6) $\dfrac{100}{120}$ (15) $\dfrac{270}{300}$ (24) $\dfrac{320}{800}$ (33) $\dfrac{450}{3000}$

(7) $\dfrac{130}{150}$ (16) $\dfrac{300}{500}$ (25) $\dfrac{1000}{1500}$ (34) $\dfrac{1500}{4000}$

(8) $\dfrac{100}{150}$ (17) $\dfrac{450}{500}$ (26) $\dfrac{800}{1500}$ (35) $\dfrac{1200}{4000}$

(9) $\dfrac{60}{150}$ (18) $\dfrac{120}{500}$ (27) $\dfrac{1250}{1500}$ (36) $\dfrac{2750}{4000}$

Fractions to tenths

Many/most syringes are graduated in tenths of a millilitre.

One tenth of a millilitre $= \frac{1}{10}$ ml
$= 0.1$ ml

WRITING AN ANSWER CORRECT TO ONE DECIMAL PLACE.

Method: If the second decimal place is *5 or more*, then ADD ONE to the first decimal place.

If the second decimal place is *less than 5*, then leave the first decimal place as it is.

EXAMPLE A(i) Write 0.76 correct to one decimal place. Rewrite the answer as tenths.

$0.7\,\textcircled{6} \approx 0.8$ $\quad \left[\begin{array}{l} \approx \text{ means} \\ \text{approximately equal} \end{array} \right]$
$0.8 = \frac{8}{10}$

EXAMPLE A(ii) Write 0.92 correct to one decimal place. Rewrite the answer as tenths.

$0.9\,\textcircled{2} \approx 0.9$
$0.9 = \frac{9}{10}$

EXAMPLE B Using decimals, change $\frac{4}{7}$ to tenths. Write the answer to the nearest tenth.

$\frac{4}{7} = 4 \div 7$ $\qquad 7)\overline{4.00}$ $\qquad \left[\begin{array}{l} \text{ignore any} \\ \text{remainder} \end{array} \right]$
$0.57 \approx 0.6$ $\qquad \quad \overline{0.57}$
$0.6 = \frac{6}{10}$ $\qquad \quad \therefore \frac{4}{7} \approx \frac{6}{10}$

EXERCISE 11

Part a
Write each number correct to one decimal place. Then
express each answer as tenths.

(1) 0·26	**(6)** 0·24	**(11)** 0·82	**(16)** 0·95
(2) 0·61	**(7)** 0·73	**(12)** 0·07	**(17)** 0·72
(3) 0·94	**(8)** 0·17	**(13)** 0·48	**(18)** 0·47
(4) 0·40	**(9)** 0·69	**(14)** 0·16	**(19)** 0·38
(5) 0·75	**(10)** 0·50	**(15)** 0·53	**(20)** 0·81

Part b
Change each vulgar fraction to a decimal, correct to one
decimal place. Then rewrite each answer as tenths.

(1) $\frac{1}{2}$	**(7)** $\frac{4}{5}$	**(13)** $\frac{5}{7}$	**(19)** $\frac{1}{9}$
(2) $\frac{1}{3}$	**(8)** $\frac{1}{6}$	**(14)** $\frac{6}{7}$	**(20)** $\frac{2}{9}$
(3) $\frac{2}{3}$	**(9)** $\frac{5}{6}$	**(15)** $\frac{1}{8}$	**(21)** $\frac{4}{9}$
(4) $\frac{1}{5}$	**(10)** $\frac{1}{7}$	**(16)** $\frac{3}{8}$	**(22)** $\frac{5}{9}$
(5) $\frac{2}{5}$	**(11)** $\frac{2}{7}$	**(17)** $\frac{5}{8}$	**(23)** $\frac{7}{9}$
(6) $\frac{3}{5}$	**(12)** $\frac{3}{7}$	**(18)** $\frac{7}{8}$	**(24)** $\frac{8}{9}$

Vulgar fraction to a decimal

METHOD   Divide the numerator (top line) by the
denominator (bottom line).

EXAMPLE A   Change $\frac{3}{8}$ to a decimal

$$8\overline{)3\cdot 000} \leftarrow \text{Write as many zeros as you need}$$
$$0\cdot 375$$

$\therefore \frac{3}{8} = 0\cdot 375$

EXAMPLE B   Change $\frac{3}{20}$ to a decimal

$$10\overline{)3\cdot}$$
$$2\overline{)0\cdot 30}$$
$$0\cdot 15$$

$\begin{bmatrix} \text{Divide by 10} \\ \text{and then 2} \\ \text{since } 10 \times 2 = 20 \end{bmatrix}$ *or* $\dfrac{3}{20} = \dfrac{15}{100}$
$$= 0\cdot 15$$

EXAMPLE C   Change $\frac{4}{25}$ to a decimal

$$5\overline{)4\cdot 0}$$
$$5\overline{)0\cdot 80}$$
$$0\cdot 16$$

$\begin{bmatrix} \text{Divide by 5} \\ \text{and then 5 again} \\ \text{since } 5 \times 5 = 25 \end{bmatrix}$ *or* $\dfrac{4}{25} = \dfrac{16}{100}$
$$= 0\cdot 16$$

EXAMPLE D   Change $\frac{4}{7}$ to a decimal
correct to 2 decimal places

$$7\overline{)4\cdot 000}$$
$$0\cdot 57①$$

$\therefore \frac{4}{7} \approx 0\cdot 57$

EXAMPLE E   Change $\frac{13}{60}$ to a decimal
correct to 3 decimal places

$$10\overline{)13\cdot}$$
$$6\overline{)1\cdot 3000}$$
$$0\cdot 216⑥$$

$\begin{bmatrix} \text{Divide by 10} \\ \text{and then 6} \\ \text{since } 10 \times 6 = 60 \end{bmatrix}$ $\therefore \dfrac{13}{60} \approx 0\cdot 217$

EXERCISE 1J

Part a
Change to a decimal.

All of these have
exact decimal
equivalents.

(1) $\dfrac{1}{2}$ (11) $\dfrac{1}{25}$

(2) $\dfrac{1}{4}$ (12) $\dfrac{7}{25}$

(3) $\dfrac{3}{4}$ (13) $\dfrac{22}{25}$

(4) $\dfrac{2}{5}$ (14) $\dfrac{1}{40}$

(5) $\dfrac{3}{5}$ (15) $\dfrac{9}{40}$

(6) $\dfrac{1}{8}$ (16) $\dfrac{11}{40}$

(7) $\dfrac{7}{8}$ (17) $\dfrac{27}{40}$

(8) $\dfrac{1}{20}$ (18) $\dfrac{1}{50}$

(9) $\dfrac{7}{20}$ (19) $\dfrac{1}{80}$

(10) $\dfrac{13}{20}$ (20) $\dfrac{19}{80}$

Part b
Change to a decimal.

Write correct to 2 decimal places. | Write correct to 3 decimal places.

(1) $\dfrac{1}{3}$ (11) $\dfrac{1}{30}$

(2) $\dfrac{2}{3}$ (12) $\dfrac{11}{30}$

(3) $\dfrac{1}{6}$ (13) $\dfrac{29}{30}$

(4) $\dfrac{5}{6}$ (14) $\dfrac{1}{60}$

(5) $\dfrac{1}{7}$ (15) $\dfrac{7}{60}$

(6) $\dfrac{3}{7}$ (16) $\dfrac{17}{60}$

(7) $\dfrac{6}{7}$ (17) $\dfrac{1}{70}$

(8) $\dfrac{1}{9}$ (18) $\dfrac{9}{70}$

(9) $\dfrac{5}{9}$ (19) $\dfrac{1}{90}$

(10) $\dfrac{8}{9}$ (20) $\dfrac{47}{90}$

Vulgar fraction to a percentage

Percentage means

PARTS IN A HUNDRED or PARTS PER HUNDRED.

EXAMPLE A   Change $\frac{7}{20}$ to a percentage

$$\frac{7}{20} = \frac{7}{\overset{}{\underset{1}{\cancel{20}}}} \times \frac{\overset{5}{\cancel{100}}}{1}\% \quad [\text{'Cancel' across by 20}]$$

$$= \frac{35}{1}\%$$

$$= 35\%$$

EXAMPLE B   Change $\frac{3}{8}$ to a percentage

$$\frac{3}{8} = \frac{3}{\overset{}{\underset{2}{\cancel{8}}}} \times \frac{\overset{25}{\cancel{100}}}{1}\% \quad [\text{'Cancel' across by 4}]$$

$$= \frac{75}{2}\%$$

$$= 37\frac{1}{2}\%$$

EXERCISE 1K   Change to a percentage.

(1) $\frac{1}{2}$	**(11)** $\frac{9}{10}$	**(21)** $\frac{7}{25}$	**(31)** $\frac{7}{8}$
(2) $\frac{1}{4}$	**(12)** $\frac{1}{20}$	**(22)** $\frac{11}{25}$	**(32)** $\frac{1}{6}$
(3) $\frac{3}{4}$	**(13)** $\frac{3}{20}$	**(23)** $\frac{13}{25}$	**(33)** $\frac{5}{6}$
(4) $\frac{1}{5}$	**(14)** $\frac{9}{20}$	**(24)** $\frac{17}{25}$	**(34)** $\frac{1}{9}$
(5) $\frac{2}{5}$	**(15)** $\frac{11}{20}$	**(25)** $\frac{19}{25}$	**(35)** $\frac{4}{9}$
(6) $\frac{3}{5}$	**(16)** $\frac{13}{20}$	**(26)** $\frac{23}{25}$	**(36)** $\frac{7}{9}$
(7) $\frac{4}{5}$	**(17)** $\frac{17}{20}$	**(27)** $\frac{1}{3}$	**(37)** $\frac{1}{40}$
(8) $\frac{1}{10}$	**(18)** $\frac{19}{20}$	**(28)** $\frac{2}{3}$	**(38)** $\frac{3}{40}$
(9) $\frac{3}{10}$	**(19)** $\frac{1}{25}$	**(29)** $\frac{1}{8}$	**(39)** $\frac{9}{40}$
(10) $\frac{7}{10}$	**(20)** $\frac{3}{25}$	**(30)** $\frac{5}{8}$	**(40)** $\frac{11}{40}$

Dilution ratios

The strength of a solution may be given as a ratio in either of two ways, e.g. '1 in 4' is equivalent to '1 to 3'. [1 to 3 may be written as 1:3]

1 in 4 means 1 part of stock solution *in* 4 parts of diluted solution.

1:3 means 1 part of stock solution added *to* 3 parts of diluent.

[DILUENT: a substance that dilutes or dissolves.]

EXAMPLE A   Change the ratio 1:5 to the form 1 *in* x

$1 + 5 = 6$ parts
$\therefore 1 : 5 = 1$ in 6

EXAMPLE B   Change the ratio 1 *in* 10 to the form 1:y

$10 - 1 = 9$ parts of diluent
$\therefore 1$ in $10 = 1:9$

EXAMPLE C   How much stock solution is present in 200 ml of diluted solution if the strength of the solution is
(a) 1 in 5   (b) 1:5?

(a)   1 in $5 = \frac{1}{5}$
$\frac{1}{5} \times 200$ ml $= 40$ ml

(b) $1:5 = 1$ in $6 = \frac{1}{6}$
$\frac{1}{6} \times 200$ ml $= 33$ ml
(to the nearest ml)

NOTE   A ratio may be written as a fraction.

EXERCISE 1 L

Part a
Change these ratios to the form 1 *in* x

(1) 1:2	**(4)** 1:10	**(7)** 1:30	**(10)** 1:200
(2) 1:5	**(5)** 1:15	**(8)** 1:50	**(11)** 1:250
(3) 1:7	**(6)** 1:25	**(9)** 1:100	**(12)** 1:500

Part b
Change these ratios to the form 1:y

(1) 1 in 2	**(4)** 1 in 7	**(7)** 1 in 20	**(10)** 1 in 50
(2) 1 in 3	**(5)** 1 in 10	**(8)** 1 in 25	**(11)** 1 in 100
(3) 1 in 5	**(6)** 1 in 15	**(9)** 1 in 40	**(12)** 1 in 200

Part c
How much stock solution is present in the given volume of diluted solution?

	Volume of diluted solution	Dilution ratios a	b	
1	100 ml	1 in 4	1:4	Calculate
2	150 ml	1 in 2	1:2	answers
3	300 ml	1 in 5	1:5	to the
4	600 ml	1 in 3	1:3	nearest
5	420 ml	1 in 6	1:6	millilitre
6	550 ml	1 in 10	1:10	
7	400 ml	1 in 3	1:3	
8	750 ml	1 in 4	1:4	
9	900 ml	1 in 6	1:6	
10	1 litre	1 in 7	1:7	
11	2 litres	1 in 8	1:8	
12	5 litres	1 in 9	1:9	

Ratio to percentage

The strength of a solution may be given as a ratio
(e.g. 1 in 5 or 1:4) or as a percentage (20%).

EXAMPLE A   Change the ratio 1 in 40 to a
percentage.

$$1 \text{ in } 40 = \frac{1}{\underset{2}{\cancel{40}}} \times \frac{\overset{5}{\cancel{100}}}{1}\% \quad [\text{'Cancel' across by 20}]$$

$$= \frac{5}{2}\% \quad \text{or } 2\cdot5\%$$

EXAMPLE B   Change 1 in 500 to a percentage.

$$1 \text{ in } 500 = \frac{1}{\underset{5}{\cancel{500}}} \times \frac{\overset{1}{\cancel{100}}}{1}\%$$

$$\begin{array}{r} 5)\overline{1\cdot000} \\ \hline 0\cdot2 \end{array}$$

$$= \frac{1}{5}\% \quad \text{or } 0\cdot2\% \quad [\text{Note answer } \textit{less than } 1\%]$$

EXAMPLE C   Change 1 in 600 to a percentage
correct to 0·01%.

$$1 \text{ in } 600 = \frac{1}{\underset{6}{\cancel{600}}} \times \frac{\overset{1}{\cancel{100}}}{1}\%$$

$$\begin{array}{r} 6)\overline{1\cdot000} \\ \hline 0\cdot16\textcircled{6} \end{array}$$

$$= \frac{1}{6}\% \quad \approx 0\cdot17\%$$

EXAMPLE D   Change 1:10 to a percentage
correct to two decimal places.

$$1:10 = 1 \text{ in } 11$$

$$= \frac{1}{11} \times \frac{100}{1}\%$$

$$\begin{array}{r} \overset{1\ \ 10}{11)\overline{100\cdot00\,0}} \\ \hline 9\cdot09\textcircled{0} \end{array}$$

$$= \frac{100}{11}\% \quad \text{or } 9\cdot09\%$$

EXERCISE 1M   Change each ratio to a percentage correct to two decimal places (where necessary).

(1) 1 in 2	**(17)** 1 in 3	**(33)** 1 in 800
(2) 1 in 4	**(18)** 1 in 6	**(34)** 1 in 900
(3) 1 in 5	**(19)** 1 in 7	**(35)** Can you see the relationship between 1 in 2, 1 in 20, 1 in 200; or 1 in 3, 1 in 30, 1 in 300, etc...?
(4) 1 in 10	**(20)** 1 in 8	
(5) 1 in 20	**(21)** 1 in 9	
(6) 1 in 25	**(22)** 1 in 12	
(7) 1 in 50	**(23)** 1 in 15	
(8) 1 in 100	**(24)** 1 in 30	
(9) 1 in 200	**(25)** 1 in 60	Now do these:
(10) 1 in 250	**(26)** 1 in 70	**(36)** 1:2
(11) 1 in 400	**(27)** 1 in 75	**(37)** 1:3
(12) 1 in 1000	**(28)** 1 in 80	**(38)** 1:5
(13) 1 in 2000	**(29)** 1 in 90	**(39)** 1:6
(14) 1 in 2500	**(30)** 1 in 300	**(40)** 1:7
(15) 1 in 5000	**(31)** 1 in 400	**(41)** 1:8
(16) 1 in 10 000	**(32)** 1 in 700	**(42)** 1:9

NOTE   A ratio may be written as a fraction or an equivalent percentage

$$\text{(e.g. 1 in 5} = \tfrac{1}{5} = 20\%).$$

Decimal fraction to vulgar fraction

EXAMPLE A   Change 0·4 to a vulgar fraction and simplify.

$$0·4 = \frac{4}{10}$$

$$= \frac{2}{5}$$

EXAMPLE B   Change 0·36 to a vulgar fraction and simplify.

$$0·36 = \frac{36}{100}$$

$$= \frac{9}{25}$$

EXERCISE 1N   Change to a vulgar fraction and simplify
where possible.

Part a

(1)	0·1	**(3)**	0·3	**(5)**	0·6	**(7)**	0·8
(2)	0·2	**(4)**	0·5	**(6)**	0·7	**(8)**	0·9

Part b

(1)	0·24	**(11)**	0·03	**(21)**	0·75	**(31)**	0·57
(2)	0·46	**(12)**	0·72	**(22)**	0·26	**(32)**	0·87
(3)	0·77	**(13)**	0·65	**(23)**	0·39	**(33)**	0·41
(4)	0·13	**(14)**	0·25	**(24)**	0·53	**(34)**	0·08
(5)	0·35	**(15)**	0·36	**(25)**	0·18	**(35)**	0·64
(6)	0·81	**(16)**	0·58	**(26)**	0·69	**(36)**	0·28
(7)	0·66	**(17)**	0·16	**(27)**	0·48	**(37)**	0·79
(8)	0·01	**(18)**	0·83	**(28)**	0·05	**(38)**	0·38
(9)	0·95	**(19)**	0·45	**(29)**	0·85	**(39)**	0·99
(10)	0·55	**(20)**	0·96	**(30)**	0·92	**(40)**	0·15

Percentage to vulgar fraction

The strength of a solution may be expressed as a percentage or as a ratio, e.g. 25% or 1 in 4 or 1 : 3. The ratio 1 in 4 can be written as a fraction $\frac{1}{4}$.

EXAMPLE A   Change 16% to a vulgar fraction.

$$16\% \quad = \frac{16}{100}$$

$$= \frac{4}{25} \quad [\text{Always simplify if possible}]$$

EXAMPLE B(i)   Change 0·3% to a vulgar fraction.

$$0\cdot3\% = \frac{0\cdot3}{100} \left[\begin{array}{l}\text{Multiply numerator} \\ \text{and denominator by 10}\end{array}\right]$$

$$= \frac{3}{1000} \quad \text{which cannot be simplified}$$

EXAMPLE B(ii)   Change 0·08% to a vulgar fraction.

$$0\cdot08\% = \frac{0\cdot08}{100} \left[\begin{array}{l}\text{Multiply numerator} \\ \text{and denominator by 100}\end{array}\right]$$

$$= \frac{8}{10\,000}$$

EXAMPLE C   Change $3\frac{1}{2}$% to a vulgar fraction.

$$3\tfrac{1}{2}\% \quad = \frac{3\frac{1}{2}}{100} \left[\begin{array}{l}\text{Multiply numerator} \\ \text{and denominator by 2}\end{array}\right]$$

$$= \frac{7}{200} \quad \text{which cannot be simplified}$$

EXERCISE 10   Change each percentage to a vulgar fraction and simplify ('cancel down') if possible.

Part a

(1) 2%	**(6)** 10%	**(11)** 35%
(2) 3%	**(7)** 12%	**(12)** 40%
(3) 4%	**(8)** 15%	**(13)** 45%
(4) 5%	**(9)** 20%	**(14)** 50%
(5) 7%	**(10)** 30%	**(15)** 90%

Part b

(1) 0·1%	**(6)** 0·7%	**(11)** 0·04%
(2) 0·2%	**(7)** 0·8%	**(12)** 0·05%
(3) 0·4%	**(8)** 0·9%	**(13)** 0·06%
(4) 0·5%	**(9)** 0·01%	**(14)** 0·07%
(5) 0·6%	**(10)** 0·02%	**(15)** 0·09%

Part c

(1) $\frac{1}{2}$%	**(3)** $2\frac{1}{2}$%	**(5)** $7\frac{1}{2}$%
(2) $1\frac{1}{2}$%	**(4)** $4\frac{1}{2}$%	**(6)** $12\frac{1}{2}$%

NOTE   A percentage may be changed to a fraction or an equivalent ratio

(e.g. **5%** = $\frac{1}{20}$ = **1 in 20**).

Multiplication of vulgar fractions

EXAMPLE A $\frac{2}{5} \times \frac{4}{7}$

$$\frac{2}{5} \times \frac{4}{7} = \frac{2 \times 4}{5 \times 7}$$

$$= \frac{8}{35} \quad \left[\begin{array}{l} \text{This fraction can} \\ \text{not be simplified} \end{array} \right]$$

EXAMPLE B $\frac{5}{8} \times \frac{7}{10}$

$$\frac{\overset{1}{\cancel{5}}}{8} \times \frac{7}{\underset{2}{\cancel{10}}} = \frac{1 \times 7}{8 \times 2} \quad \left[\begin{array}{l} \text{Note cancelling} \\ \text{across by 5} \end{array} \right]$$

$$= \frac{7}{16}$$

EXAMPLE C $\frac{4}{9} \times \frac{21}{5}$

$$\frac{4}{\underset{3}{\cancel{9}}} \times \frac{\overset{7}{\cancel{21}}}{5} = \frac{4 \times 7}{3 \times 5} \quad \left[\begin{array}{l} \text{Note cancelling} \\ \text{across by 3} \end{array} \right]$$

$$= \frac{28}{15}$$

$$= 1\frac{13}{15} \quad [\text{Answers may be greater than one}]$$

EXAMPLE D $\frac{9}{10} \times \frac{8}{15}$

$$\frac{\overset{3}{\cancel{9}}}{\underset{5}{\cancel{10}}} \times \frac{\overset{4}{\cancel{8}}}{\underset{5}{\cancel{15}}} = \frac{3 \times 4}{5 \times 5} \quad \left[\begin{array}{l} \text{Note cancelling across} \\ \text{by 3 and by 2} \end{array} \right]$$

$$= \frac{12}{25}$$

EXERCISE 1P   Multiply. Simplify where possible.

(1) $\frac{1}{2} \times \frac{2}{5}$

(2) $\frac{1}{3} \times \frac{5}{8}$

(3) $\frac{2}{3} \times \frac{5}{6}$

(4) $\frac{1}{4} \times \frac{2}{3}$

(5) $\frac{3}{4} \times \frac{20}{9}$

(6) $\frac{1}{5} \times \frac{3}{10}$

(7) $\frac{2}{5} \times \frac{3}{2}$

(8) $\frac{3}{5} \times \frac{3}{4}$

(9) $\frac{4}{5} \times \frac{25}{24}$

(10) $\frac{1}{6} \times \frac{9}{10}$

(11) $\frac{5}{6} \times \frac{8}{15}$

(12) $\frac{1}{7} \times \frac{7}{18}$

(13) $\frac{2}{7} \times \frac{11}{12}$

(14) $\frac{3}{7} \times \frac{1}{20}$

(15) $\frac{4}{7} \times \frac{5}{3}$

(16) $\frac{5}{7} \times \frac{12}{25}$

(17) $\frac{6}{7} \times \frac{5}{24}$

(18) $\frac{1}{8} \times \frac{1}{2}$

(19) $\frac{3}{8} \times \frac{12}{5}$

(20) $\frac{5}{8} \times \frac{9}{20}$

(21) $\frac{7}{8} \times \frac{8}{7}$

(22) $\frac{1}{9} \times \frac{1}{15}$

(23) $\frac{2}{9} \times \frac{7}{4}$

(24) $\frac{4}{9} \times \frac{5}{12}$

(25) $\frac{5}{9} \times \frac{21}{25}$

(26) $\frac{7}{9} \times \frac{9}{16}$

(27) $\frac{8}{9} \times \frac{1}{6}$

(28) $\frac{1}{10} \times \frac{15}{8}$

(29) $\frac{3}{10} \times \frac{4}{9}$

(30) $\frac{7}{10} \times \frac{2}{7}$

(31) $\frac{9}{10} \times \frac{15}{16}$

(32) $\frac{1}{11} \times \frac{11}{18}$

(33) $\frac{1}{12} \times \frac{1}{30}$

(34) $\frac{5}{12} \times \frac{7}{30}$

(35) $\frac{7}{12} \times \frac{9}{40}$

(36) $\frac{11}{12} \times \frac{33}{40}$

Division by a vulgar fraction

Drug dosage and dilution calculations often involve division by a vulgar fraction.

METHOD   To divide by a vulgar fraction, invert the divisor and then multiply.
[Note: The DIVISOR is the number you are dividing by.]

or   To divide by a vulgar fraction, multiply by its reciprocal.
[Note: The reciprocal of $\frac{a}{b}$ is $\frac{b}{a}$]

EXAMPLE A $\frac{2}{3} \div \frac{4}{5}$

$$\frac{2}{3} \div \frac{4}{5} = \frac{\overset{1}{2}}{3} \times \frac{5}{\underset{2}{4}} \quad [\text{'Cancelling' across by 2}]$$

$$= \frac{5}{6}$$

EXAMPLE B $\frac{9}{10} \div \frac{6}{7}$

$$\frac{9}{10} \div \frac{6}{7} = \frac{\overset{3}{9}}{10} \times \frac{7}{\underset{2}{6}} \quad [\text{'Cancelling' across by 3}]$$

$$= \frac{21}{20}$$

$$= 1\tfrac{1}{20}$$

EXERCISE 1Q   Divide. Simplify where possible.

(1) $\frac{1}{2} \div \frac{3}{4}$

(2) $\frac{1}{2} \div \frac{1}{3}$

(3) $\frac{1}{3} \div \frac{1}{4}$

(4) $\frac{1}{3} \div \frac{5}{9}$

(5) $\frac{2}{3} \div \frac{1}{6}$

(6) $\frac{2}{3} \div \frac{4}{9}$

(7) $\frac{1}{4} \div \frac{1}{2}$

(8) $\frac{1}{4} \div \frac{4}{5}$

(9) $\frac{3}{4} \div \frac{5}{6}$

(10) $\frac{3}{4} \div \frac{1}{5}$

(11) $\frac{1}{5} \div \frac{1}{3}$

(12) $\frac{2}{5} \div \frac{3}{5}$

(13) $\frac{3}{5} \div \frac{9}{10}$

(14) $\frac{4}{5} \div \frac{2}{3}$

(15) $\frac{1}{6} \div \frac{7}{9}$

(16) $\frac{5}{6} \div \frac{2}{5}$

(17) $\frac{1}{7} \div \frac{1}{8}$

(18) $\frac{2}{7} \div \frac{4}{5}$

(19) $\frac{3}{7} \div \frac{9}{10}$

(20) $\frac{4}{7} \div \frac{1}{3}$

(21) $\frac{5}{7} \div \frac{10}{3}$

(22) $\frac{6}{7} \div \frac{3}{4}$

(23) $\frac{1}{8} \div \frac{7}{8}$

(24) $\frac{3}{8} \div \frac{9}{10}$

(25) $\frac{5}{8} \div \frac{5}{6}$

(26) $\frac{7}{8} \div \frac{1}{2}$

(27) $\frac{1}{9} \div \frac{1}{5}$

(28) $\frac{2}{9} \div \frac{2}{3}$

(29) $\frac{4}{9} \div \frac{1}{6}$

(30) $\frac{5}{9} \div \frac{5}{8}$

(31) $\frac{7}{9} \div \frac{7}{10}$

(32) $\frac{8}{9} \div \frac{2}{3}$

(33) $\frac{1}{10} \div \frac{1}{7}$

(34) $\frac{3}{10} \div \frac{5}{6}$

(35) $\frac{7}{10} \div \frac{7}{8}$

(36) $\frac{9}{10} \div \frac{3}{5}$

Converting units of length

EXAMPLE A   Using the conversion tables given opposite, change a height of 5′ 7″ to centimetres (to the nearest cm).

5 feet   = 152·4 cm
7 inches =   17·8 cm   +
              170·2 cm

Answer: 170 cm (to nearest cm)

EXAMPLE B   Change a child's height of 3′ 8″ to centimetres (to the nearest cm).

3 feet   =   91·4 cm
8 inches =   20·3 cm   +
              111·7 cm

Answer: 112 cm (to nearest cm)

Feet	cm	Inches	cm
1	30·5	1	2·5
2	61·0	2	5·1
3	91·4	3	7·6
4	121·9	4	10·2
5	152·4	5	12·7
6	182·9	6	15·2
7	213·4	7	17·8
8	243·8	8	20·3
		9	22·9
		10	25·4
		11	27·9

Lengths in cm
correct to 0·1 cm

EXERCISE 1R   Using the given conversion tables,
change the following heights from feet and inches to
centimetres (to the nearest cm).

(1) 2′ 8″   **(6)** 4′ 3″   **(11)** 5′ 2″

(2) 2′ 11″   **(7)** 4′ 10″   **(12)** 6′ 1″

(3) 3′ 7″   **(8)** 4′ 6″   **(13)** 6′ 5″

(4) 3′ 4″   **(9)** 5′ 5″   **(14)** 6′ 8″

(5) 3′ 11″   **(10)** 5′ 9″   **(15)** 7′ 2″

Converting units of weight

EXAMPLE A Using the conversion tables (given opposite and below), change a weight of 6 stone 10 lb to kilograms (to the nearest kg).

$$
\begin{array}{ll}
6 \text{ stone} & = 38 \cdot 1 \text{ kg} \\
10 \text{ lb} & = \underline{4 \cdot 5 \text{ kg}} \\
& 42 \cdot 6 \text{ kg}
\end{array} \Big+
$$

Answer: 43 kg (to nearest kg)

EXAMPLE B Change a weight of 15 stone 4 lb to kilograms (to the nearest kg).

$$
\begin{array}{ll}
15 \text{ stone} & = 95 \cdot 3 \text{ kg} \\
4 \text{ lb} & = \underline{1 \cdot 8 \text{ kg}} \\
& 97 \cdot 1 \text{ kg}
\end{array} \Big+
$$

Answer: 97 kg (to nearest kg)

Pounds	1	2	3	4	5	6	7
kg	0·5	0·9	1·4	1·8	2·3	2·7	3·2

Pounds	8	9	10	11	12	13	
kg	3·6	4·1	4·5	5·0	5·4	5·9	

EXERCISE 1S   Change the following weights to kilograms (to the nearest kg).

Stone	Kilogram
1	6·4
2	12·7
3	19·1
4	25·4
5	31·8
6	38·1
7	44·5
8	50·8
9	57·2
10	63·5
11	69·9
12	76·2
13	82·6
14	88·9
15	95·3
16	101·6
17	108·0
18	114·3
19	120·7
20	127·0

Weights in kg
correct to 0·1 kg

(1)   3 st 10 lb
(2)   4 st 3 lb
(3)   5 st 11 lb
(4)   6 st 4 lb
(5)   7 st 12 lb
(6)   8 st 9 lb
(7)   9 st 2 lb
(8) 10 st 13 lb
(9) 11 st 5 lb
(10) 12 st 1 lb
(11) 13 st 3 lb
(12) 14 st 6 lb
(13) 15 st 5 lb
(14) 16 st 7 lb
(15) 17 st 8 lb
(16) 18 st 7 lb
(17) 19 st 9 lb
(18) 20 st 1 lb

EXERCISE 15: Change the following weights to
kilogram (to 1 decimal place)

Stone	Kilogram	
1	8·4	(1)
2	13·7	(2)
3	19·1	(3)
4	25·2	(4)
5	31·8	(5)
6	38·1	(6)
7	44·5	(7)
8	50·8	(8)
9	57·2	(9)
10	63·5	(10)
11	69·9	(11)
12	76·2	(12)
13	82·6	(13)
14	88·9	(14)
15	95·3	(15)
16	101·6	(16)
17	108·0	(17)
18	114·3	(18)
19	120·7	
20	127·0	

Weights to kg
correct to 0·1 kg

2. Drug dosages for injection

Correct measurement of drug dosages for injection is most important. An overdose can be dangerous: too low a dose may result in a drug being ineffective.

The number of decimal places in each answer should match the graduations on the syringe being used. Syringes with a capacity of more than 1 ml are usually graduated in tenths or fifths of a ml: so for volumes *greater* than 1 ml calculate answers correct to *one* decimal place. Syringes with a capacity of 1 ml or less are often graduated in hundredths of a ml: so for volumes *less* than 1 ml calculate answers to *two* decimal places.

Check that stock strength and the strength required are given in the *same* unit in a particular problem (i.e. *both* strengths in grams or milligrams or micrograms or millimoles).

Be VERY CAREFUL when working in MICROGRAMS: write the word 'micrograms' in full to avoid any confusion.

EXAMPLE 1 A patient is ordered cortisone 40 mg, I.M.I. Ampoules contain cortisone 50 mg in 2 ml. Calculate the volume required for injection.

$$\frac{\text{Volume}}{\text{required}} = \frac{\text{Strength required}}{\text{stock strength}} \times \left(\begin{array}{c} \text{Volume of} \\ \text{stock solution} \end{array} \right)$$

$$= \frac{40\,\text{mg}}{50\,\text{mg}} \times 2\,\text{ml}$$

$$= \frac{40}{50} \times \frac{2}{1}\,\text{ml}$$

$$= \frac{8}{5}\,\text{ml} \quad \text{or } 1\cdot6\,\text{ml}$$

EXAMPLE 2 An injection of digoxin 175 micrograms is ordered. Stock on hand is digoxin 500 micrograms in 2 ml. What volume of stock should be given? [N.B. MICROGRAMS]

$$\frac{\text{Volume}}{\text{required}} = \frac{\text{Strength required}}{\text{Stock strength}} \times \left(\begin{array}{c} \text{Volume of} \\ \text{stock solution} \end{array} \right)$$

$$= \frac{175\,\text{micrograms}}{500\,\text{micrograms}} \times 2\,\text{ml}$$

$$= \frac{175}{500} \times \frac{2}{1}\,\text{ml}$$

$$= \frac{7}{10}\,\text{ml} \quad \text{or } 0\cdot7\,\text{ml}$$

EXAMPLE 3. Potassium chloride 20 mmol, I.M.I. is ordered. Stock solution contains 25 mmol/10 ml. What volume should be drawn up?

$$\frac{\text{Volume}}{\text{required}} = \frac{\text{Strength required}}{\text{Stock strength}} \times \left(\begin{array}{c} \text{Volume of} \\ \text{stock solution} \end{array} \right)$$

$$= \frac{20\,\text{mmol}}{25\,\text{mmol}} \times 10\,\text{ml}$$

$$= \frac{20}{25} \times \frac{10}{1}\,\text{ml}$$

$$= 8\,\text{ml}$$

EXERCISE 2A

1. An injection of morphine 8 mg is required. Ampoules on hand contain 10 mg in 1 ml. What volume is drawn up for injection?

2. Digoxin ampoules on hand contain 500 micrograms in 2 ml. What volume is needed to give 350 micrograms?

3. A patient is ordered 16 mmol of potassium chloride. Stock solution contains potassium chloride 25 mmol in 10 ml. What volume is needed?

4. A patient is to be given erythromycin 120 mg by injection. Stock vials contain 300 mg/10 ml. Calculate the required volume.

5. Stock heparin has a strength of 5000 units per ml. What volume must be drawn up to give 6500 units?

6. Pethidine 85 mg is to be given I.M., as premedication. Stock ampoules contain pethidine 100 mg in 2 ml. Calculate volume of stock required.

7. A patient is to receive an injection of gentamicin 60 mg, I.M. Ampoules on hand contain 80 mg/2 ml. Calculate volume required.

EXERCISE 2B

1. Kantrex 500 mg is ordered. Stock on hand contains 1 gram in 3 ml. What volume is required?

2. A patient is to receive an injection of erythromycin 160 mg. Stock ampoules contain 100 mg in 2 ml. Calculate the volume to be drawn up for injection.

3. How much morphine solution must be withdrawn for a 9 mg dose if a stock ampoule contains 15 mg in 1 ml?

4. A patient is ordered 2 megaunits of crystalline penicillin. Stock is 5 megaunits in 10 ml. Calculate the volume that is needed.

5. Heparin is available at a strength of 1000 units/ml. What volume is needed to give 800 units?

6. Phenobarbitone 40 mg has been ordered. Stock ampoules contain 200 mg/ml. What volume should be given?

7. A patient is ordered pethidine 65 mg as premedication. Stock ampoules of pethidine contain 100 mg in 2 ml. Calculate the volume to be drawn up for injection.

EXERCISE 2C   Calculate the volume of stock to be drawn up for injection.

1. A patient is prescribed erythromycin 80 mg by I.M.I. Stock ampoules contain 100 mg/2 ml.

2. Pethidine 60 mg is ordered. Stock ampoules contain 100 mg in 2 ml.

3. An adult is ordered Omnopon 24 mg, premedication. On hand are ampoules containing 20 mg/ml.

4. A patient is ordered Bicillin 150 000 units. On hand is Bicillin 1·2 megaunits in 2 ml.

5. Cortisone 60 mg is required. Available stock contains 125 mg in 5 ml.

6. An adult patient with TB is to be given 3000 mg of streptomycin, I.M.I. Stock ampoules contain 5 grams in 5 ml.

7. Digoxin ampoules on hand contain 500 micrograms in 2 ml. Digoxin 150 micrograms is ordered.

8. Stock Calciparine contains 25 000 units in 1 ml. 15 000 units of Calciparine are ordered.

9. Penicillin 400 000 units is ordered. Stock ampoules contain 1 meganunit in 2 ml.

**NOTE   1 megaunit = 1 million units.
The symbol for megaunit is Mu.**

EXERCISE 2D   Calculate the amount of stock solution
to be drawn up for injection. Give answers greater than
1 ml correct to one decimal place; answers less than 1 ml
correct to 2 decimal places.
If the next decimal place is a 5, add one to the previous
digit.

1. Ordered : erythromycin 200 mg
      Stock : 300 mg in 10 ml

2. Ordered : morphine 20 mg
      Stock : 15 mg in 1 ml

3. Ordered : atropine 0·5 mg
      Stock : 0·6 mg in 1 ml

4. Ordered : atropine 800 micrograms
      Stock : 1·2 mg in 1 ml

5. Ordered : Bicillin 400 000 units
      Stock : 1·2 Mu/2 ml

6. Ordered : streptomycin 850 mg
      Stock : 2 grams per ml

7. Ordered : potassium chloride 18 mmol
      Stock : 25 mmol/10 ml

8. Ordered : heparin 1750 units
      Stock : 1000 units per ml

9. Ordered : scopolamine 0·25 mg
      Stock : 0·4 mg/2 ml

EXERCISE 2E   Calculate the volume of stock required.

	Ordered		Stock ampoule
1	Morphine	9 mg	15 mg/ml
2	Calciparine	7000 units	25 000 U. in 1 ml
3	Cryst. penicillin	3·5 mega-units	5 megaunits in 10 ml
4	Heparin	3000 units	5000 U./ml
5	Phenobarb	70 mg	200 mg/ml
6	Pethidine	80 mg	100 mg/2 ml
7	Scopolamine	0·24 mg	0·4 mg/2 ml
8	Digoxin	200 micro-grams	500 micrograms in 2 ml
9	Cortisone	75 mg	125 mg in 5 ml
10	Cortisone	90 mg	250 mg in 10 ml
11	Streptomycin	800 mg	1 gram in 5 ml
12	Cryst. penicillin	150 000 units	1 million units in 2 ml
13	Chloramphenicol	75 mg	250 mg in 5 ml
14	Methicillin	1500 mg	1 gram in 5 ml
15	Morphine	7·5 mg	10 mg in 1 ml
16	Methicillin	2100 mg	1 g/3 ml
17	Omnopon	34 mg	20 mg in 1 ml
18	Dexamethasone	3 mg	4 mg/ml
19	Bicillin	900 000 U.	1·2 Mu/2 ml
20	Largactil	18 mg	25 mg/ml

3. Dosages of tablets and mixtures

Drugs may be administered by injection, by I.V. infusion, or orally. Oral dosages may be in the form of tablets, capsules or mixtures.

Many mixtures are *suspensions*. These must be shaken thoroughly, in order to obtain the correct stock strength, before measuring out the required volume.

EXAMPLE 1   How many 30 mg tablets of phenobarb should be given for a dose of phenobarb 45 mg?

$$\text{Volume required} = \frac{\text{Strength required}}{\text{Stock strength}} \times \left(\text{Volume of stock solution} \right)$$

$$= \frac{45\,\text{mg}}{30\,\text{mg}} \times 1 \text{ tablet}$$

$$= 1\tfrac{1}{2} \text{ tablets}$$

EXAMPLE 2   A patient is ordered 0·25 mg of digoxin, orally. The digoxin available is in tablets containing 125 micrograms. How many such tablets should the patient receive?

CHANGE BOTH STRENGTHS TO THE SAME UNIT.

$0\cdot25\,\text{mg} = 250$ micrograms

$$\therefore \text{Volume required} = \frac{\text{Strength required}}{\text{Stock strength}} \times \left(\text{Volume of stock solution} \right)$$

$$= \frac{250\,\text{micrograms}}{125\,\text{micrograms}} \times 1 \text{ tablet}$$

$$= 2 \text{ tablets}$$

NOTE   (a) In the case of tablets, 'Volume required' refers to the number of tablets;

(b) Some answers may be less than one tablet (e.g. $\tfrac{1}{4}$, $\tfrac{1}{2}$ or $\tfrac{3}{4}$ tablet).

EXERCISE 3A

1. A patient is ordered Pensig 375 mg, orally. Stock on hand is 125 mg tablets. Calculate the number of tablets required.

2. How many 30 mg tablets of codeine are needed for a dose of 0·06 grams?

3. A patient is ordered penicillin 375 mg, orally. In the ward are 250 mg tablets. How many tablets should be given?

4. Ordered: codeine 15 mg, orally. Stock on hand: codeine tablets, 30 mg. How many tablets should the patient take?

5. 625 mg of penicillin is required. On hand are tablets of strength 250 mg. How many tablets should be given?

6. A patient is prescribed 75 mg of soluble aspirin. On hand are 300 mg tablets. What number should be given?

7. 450 mg of soluble aspirin is ordered. Stock on hand is 300 mg tablets. How many tablets should the patient receive?

EXAMPLE 3   600 mg of chloral hydrate is to be given orally as a sedative. Stock mixture contains 300 mg/5 ml. Calculate the volume of mixture to be given.

$$\text{Volume required} = \frac{\text{Strength required}}{\text{Stock strength}} \times \left(\text{Volume of stock solution} \right)$$

$$= \frac{600\,\text{mg}}{300\,\text{mg}} \times 5\,\text{ml}$$

$$= \frac{600}{300} \times \frac{5}{1}\,\text{ml}$$

$$= 10\,\text{ml}$$

EXAMPLE 4   A patient is ordered 800 mg of penicillin, orally. Stock mixture on hand has a strength of 250 mg/5 ml. Calculate the volume required.

$$\text{Volume required} = \frac{\text{Strength required}}{\text{Stock strength}} \times \left(\text{Volume of stock solution} \right)$$

$$= \frac{800\,\text{mg}}{250\,\text{mg}} \times 5\,\text{ml}$$

$$= \frac{800}{250} \times \frac{5}{1}\,\text{ml}$$

$$= 16\,\text{ml}$$

EXERCISE 3B   In each example, you are given the prescribed dosage and the strength of stock mixture on hand.
　　Calculate the volume to be given.

1.   Ordered: Pensig 500 mg
On hand: syrup 125 mg/5 ml

2.   Ordered: chloral hydrate 1500 mg
On hand: mixture 1 gram/10 ml

3.   Ordered: chloramphenicol 750 mg
On hand: suspension 125 mg/5 ml

4.   Ordered: sulphadimidine 2 grams
On hand: mixture 500 mg/5 ml

5.   Ordered: erythromycin 1250 mg
On hand: suspension 250 mg/5 ml

6.   Ordered: aspirin 900 mg
On hand: mixture 150 mg in 5 ml

7.   Ordered: penicillin 1000 mg
On hand: mixture 250 mg/5 ml

8.   Ordered: Largactil 35 mg
On hand: syrup 25 mg/5 ml

9.   Ordered: penicillin 1200 mg
On hand: mixture 250 mg/5 ml

10.   Ordered: erythromycin 800 mg
On hand: mixture 125 mg/5 ml

4. Dilution and strengths of solutions

Strengths of solutions may be stated in grams per litre, mg/ml, as ratio strengths, or as percentage strengths. Every ratio strength has an equivalent percentage strength, and vice-versa.

Most solutions are stored in concentrated form in order to save storage space. The concentrated solution is then diluted before use.

The same substance may be used at different strengths for different purposes.

REMEMBER

Percentage means parts per hundred parts.

e.g.   3% = 3 parts per hundred parts
$$= \frac{3}{100} \quad \text{(or 3 in 100)}.$$

EXAMPLE 1 **Calculate the percentage strength when 2 ml of disinfectant concentrate is made up to one litre with water.**

$$\text{One litre} = 1000\,\text{ml}$$

$$\text{Ratio strength} = \frac{2\,\text{ml}}{1000\,\text{ml}} = \frac{2}{1000}$$

$$\therefore \text{Percentage strength} = \frac{2}{1000} \times \frac{100}{1}\% = 0 \cdot 2\%$$

EXAMPLE 2 **A 2·5% sodium hypochlorite solution is to be used to bathe a wound. Express 2·5% as a ratio strength.**

$$2 \cdot 5\% = \frac{2 \cdot 5}{100} \left[\begin{array}{l} \text{Multiply numerator} \\ \text{and denominator by 10} \end{array} \right]$$

$$= \frac{25}{1000}$$

$$= \frac{1}{40} \text{ (or 1 in 40)}$$

EXAMPLE 3 **Calculate the percentage strength of the solution when 10 g of silver nitrate is dissolved in 200 ml of water.**

200 ml of water weighs 200 grams

$$\text{Ratio strength} = \frac{10\,\text{g}}{200\,\text{g}} = \frac{10}{200}$$

$$\therefore \text{Percentage strength} = \frac{10}{200} \times \frac{100}{1}\% = 5\%$$

Note that this is not strictly correct as the 10 g of silver nitrate makes the weight of the *solution* 210 grams. However, the method is sufficiently accurate for practical purposes, and is used when a *solid* is dissolved in a liquid.

EXERCISE 4A

1. Find the ratio strength of a solution when (a) 2 ml
   (b) 20 ml (c) 200 ml of pure substance is made up to
   2 litres with water.

2. Change the following percentage strengths to ratio
   strengths:
   (a) 50% (b) 25% (c) 20% (d) 10% (e) 5%
   (f) $2\frac{1}{2}$% (g) 2% (h) 0·5% (i) 0·2% (j) 0·1%.

3. Find (a) the ratio strength (b) the percentage
   strength of a solution after 15 ml of pure substance is
   mixed with 360 ml of water.

4. Find (a) the ratio strength (b) the percentage
   strength of the solution when 10 ml of concentrated
   disinfectant is made up to 200 ml with water.

5. A sodium hypochlorite solution (Milton) has a
   strength of 1 in 80. Express this as a percentage
   strength.

6. Chlorhexidine is used as a 1 : 2000 solution for a
   general antiseptic; 1 : 5000 for douches. Change
   (a) 1 : 2000 (b) 1 : 5000 to percentages.

7. Calculate the percentage strength of the solution
   when 15 grams of dextrose are dissolved in 600 ml of
   water.

EXAMPLE 4 A patient is to have a leg bathed in sterile normal saline. Four litres of normal saline solution (0·9%) are to be prepared. What volume of stock 18% saline must be used? What volume of water?

$$\left(\begin{array}{c}\text{Amount of}\\\text{stock}\\\text{required}\end{array}\right) = \frac{\text{Strength required}}{\text{Stock strength}} \times \left(\begin{array}{c}\text{Total volume}\\\text{required}\end{array}\right)$$

$$= \frac{0·9\%}{18\%} \times 4 \text{ litres}$$

$$= \frac{0·9}{18} \times \frac{4000}{1} \text{ ml}$$

$$= \frac{9}{180} \times \frac{4000}{1} \text{ ml}$$

$$= 200 \text{ ml}$$

Answer: 200 ml 18% saline, 3800 ml water

EXAMPLE 5 3 ml of 0·2% salbutamol is to be given by way of a nebulizer. Stock salbutamol has a strength of 0·5%. Calculate the required amount of (a) salbutamol (b) water.

$$\left(\begin{array}{c}\text{Amount of}\\\text{stock}\\\text{required}\end{array}\right) = \frac{\text{Strength required}}{\text{Stock strength}} \times \left(\begin{array}{c}\text{Total volume}\\\text{required}\end{array}\right)$$

$$= \frac{0·2\%}{0·5\%} \times 3 \text{ ml}$$

$$= \frac{0·2}{0·5} \times \frac{3}{1} \text{ ml}$$

$$= \frac{2}{5} \times \frac{3}{1} \text{ ml}$$

$$= 1·2 \text{ ml}$$

Answer: 1·2 ml 0·5% salbutamol, 1·8 ml water

EXERCISE 4B   Calculate the required amount of
(i) stock solution (ii) distilled water to make the
following solutions:

1. (a) One litre (b) 2 litres (c) 1·2 litres of normal
    saline (0·9%) from 18% saline.

2. (a) 500 ml (b) 750 ml (c) 2½ litres of normal saline
    (0·9%) from 4·5% saline.

3. 200 ml of cetrimide 1% from concentrated cetrimide
    40%.

4. Half a litre of cetrimide 1% from concentrated
    cetrimide 40%.

5. 30 ml of cocaine solution 1% from cocaine 2%.

6. 0·2 litres of cocaine solution 1% from cocaine 2%.

7. 4 ml of 0·3% salbutamol from 0·5% salbutamol.

8. 6 ml of 0·3% salbutamol from 0·5% salbutamol.

9. 500 ml of 1% hypochlorite solution from 10%
    hypochlorite solution.

10. One litre of 2½% hypochlorite solution from 10%
    hypochlorite solution.

EXAMPLE 6   600 ml of lotion, strength 1 in 80, is to be prepared from stock lotion of strength 1 in 20. How much stock lotion is needed? How much water?

$$\begin{pmatrix} \text{Amount of} \\ \text{stock} \\ \text{required} \end{pmatrix} = \frac{\text{Strength required}}{\text{Stock strength}} \times \begin{pmatrix} \text{Total volume} \\ \text{required} \end{pmatrix}$$

$$= \frac{1 \text{ in } 80}{1 \text{ in } 20} \times 600 \text{ ml}$$

STUDY THIS CALCULATION CAREFULLY

$$= \frac{1}{80} \div \frac{1}{20} \times \frac{600}{1} \text{ ml}$$

$$= \frac{1}{80} \times \frac{20}{1} \times \frac{600}{1} \text{ ml}$$

$$= 150 \text{ ml}$$

Answer: Stock 150 ml, water 450 ml

EXAMPLE 7   1½ litres of aqueous chlorhexidine 1 : 5000 is required for a douche. Stock solution is 2% chlorhexidine. Calculate the required amount of (a) stock (b) distilled water.

$$\begin{pmatrix} \text{Amount of} \\ \text{stock} \\ \text{required} \end{pmatrix} = \frac{\text{Strength required}}{\text{Stock strength}} \times \begin{pmatrix} \text{Total volume} \\ \text{required} \end{pmatrix}$$

$$= \frac{1 : 5000}{2\%} \times 1\tfrac{1}{2} \text{ litres}$$

STUDY THIS CALCULATION CAREFULLY

$$= \frac{1}{5000} \div \frac{2}{100} \times \frac{1500}{1} \text{ ml}$$

$$= \frac{1}{5000} \times \frac{100}{2} \times \frac{1500}{1} \text{ ml}$$

$$= 15 \text{ ml}$$

Answer: Stock 15 ml, water 1485 ml

EXERCISE 4C   Calculate the amount of (i) stock solution (ii) distilled water to make the following solutions:

1.   One litre of lotion, strength 1 in 50, from stock lotion of strength 1 in 10.

2. $1\frac{1}{2}$ litres of lotion, strength 1 in 150, from stock lotion of strength 1 in 25.

3.   500 ml of an antiseptic solution of chlorhexidine 1–2000 from stock chlorhexidine of strength 1–1000.

4.   1·5 litres of chlorhexidine 1 in 2000 from stock chlorhexidine 1 in 1000.

5.   600 ml of chlorhexidine 1 in 5000 from stock chlorhexidine 1 in 1000.

6.   Three litres of 1–5000 solution from stock solution 0·1%.

7.   2·5 litres of 0·05% solution from stock on hand, diluted 1–100.

8.   Two litres of 1–10 000 strength solution from stock solution 0·5%.

9.   700 ml of aqueous chlorhexidine 1 : 2000 from 5% stock solution.

10.   0·8 litre of 2% solution from stock solution of strength 1 in 25.

EXAMPLE 8 300 ml of Eusol 1 in 20 is to be prepared from _pure_ Eusol. How much pure Eusol is required? How much water must be added?

$$\begin{pmatrix} \text{Amount of} \\ \text{stock} \\ \text{required} \end{pmatrix} = \frac{\text{Strength required}}{\text{Stock strength}} \times \begin{pmatrix} \text{Total volume} \\ \text{required} \end{pmatrix}$$

$$= \frac{1 \text{ in } 20}{1 \text{ in } 1} \times 300 \text{ ml}$$

$$= \frac{1}{20} \times \frac{300}{1} \text{ ml}$$

$$= 15 \text{ ml}$$

Answer: Eusol 15 ml, water 285 ml

EXAMPLE 9 What volume of _pure_ Savlon is needed to prepare 1½ litres of a 2% solution?

$$\begin{pmatrix} \text{Amount of} \\ \text{stock} \\ \text{required} \end{pmatrix} = \frac{\text{Strength required}}{\text{Stock strength}} \times \begin{pmatrix} \text{Total volume} \\ \text{required} \end{pmatrix}$$

$$= \frac{2\%}{100\%} \times 1\tfrac{1}{2} \text{ litres}$$

$$= \frac{2}{100} \times \frac{1500}{1} \text{ ml} \quad \begin{bmatrix} \text{Percentage signs} \\ \text{cancels out} \end{bmatrix}$$

$$= 30 \text{ ml}$$

Answer: Savlon 30 ml

EXERCISE 4D   What quantity of PURE stock is required to make up the following solutions? How much water must be added?

[Remember that PURE stock has a strength of ONE. This may be written as just 1 *or* 1 in 1 *or* $\frac{1}{1}$ *or* 100%]

1. 800 ml of 5% solution.

2. 1·5 litres of 10% solution.

3. Five litres of 1% chlorhexidine solution.

4. $2\frac{1}{2}$ litres of 10% chlorhexidine solution.

5. One litre of 5% Savlon solution.

6. 1·2 litres of $2\frac{1}{2}$% Savlon solution.

7. 350 ml of 1% Salvon solution.

8. One litre of thymol 1–8 solution.

9. 300 ml of thymol 1–8 solution.

10. 100 ml of Eusol solution 1–16.

NOTE: In these examples, percentage strength is generally used to denote grams of solute per 100 ml of water (since 100 ml of water weighs 100 grams).

EXAMPLE 10: What weight of sodium bicarbonate is needed to prepare 1500 ml of a 5% solution to be used as a mouthwash?

5% of 1500 ml = 5% of 1500 grams
[since 1500 ml water weighs 1500 g]

$$= \frac{5}{100} \times \frac{1500}{1} g$$

$$= 75g$$

Answer: 75 g of sodium bicarbonate.

EXAMPLE 11 What volume of 0·5% salbutamol solution contains 20 mg of salbutamol?

$$0·5\% \text{ Salbutamol} = 0·5 \text{ g per } 100 \text{ g water}$$

$$= 0·5 \text{ g per } 100 \text{ ml}$$

$$= 500 \text{ mg per } 100 \text{ ml}$$

$$\therefore \text{Volume required} = \frac{\text{Strength required}}{\text{Stock strength}} \times \left(\begin{array}{c} \text{Volume of} \\ \text{stock solution} \end{array} \right)$$

$$= \frac{20 \text{ mg}}{500 \text{ mg}} \times 100 \text{ ml}$$

$$= \frac{20}{500} \times \frac{100}{1} \text{ ml}$$

$$= 4 \text{ ml}$$

EXERCISE 4E

1. How many milligrams of Largactil are present in 2 ml of 5% solution?

2. What weight of salbutamol is present in 10 ml of 0·5 solution?

3. How much dextrose is dissolved in:
   (a) 600 ml of 4% solution
   (b) $1\frac{1}{2}$ litres of 4% solution
   (c) Half a litre of 2% solution?

4. How many grams of sodium bicarbonate are needed to make:
   (a) 2 litres of a 5% solution
   (b) 3 litres of a $2\frac{1}{2}$% solution?
   (c) 1 litre of an 8·4% solution?

5. What weight of silver nitrate is dissolved in 300 ml of 5% solution?

6. What volume of *pure* ammonia is contained in a bottle of
   (a) 250 ml of 40% ammonia solution
   (b) 500 ml of 25% ammonia solution?

7. Express as percentage strengths:
   (a) 50 mg of solute per ml of water
   (b) 15 mg of solute per ml of water
   (c) 2 g of solute per litre of water.

8. What volume of 25% mannitol solution contains 20 g of mannitol?

9. What volume of 1% xylocaine solution contains 0·15 g of xylocaine?

5. Drip rates

This chapter deals with the arithmetic of drip rates for I.V. infusion.

The fluid being infused passes from a flask (or similar container) into a drip chamber.

A drip chamber has a *fixed* drop size and an *adjustable* rate of flow.

There are two main types of drip chamber in general use: one type breaks the fluid into 15 drops per ml, the other produces 60 drops per ml (microdrip).

NOTE: If the answer to a drip rate calculation is a mixed number, then use the *next whole number* for practical purposes (and to ensure that the infusion is completed in the given time).

e.g. $18\frac{3}{4}$ drops/min $\Rightarrow$ 19 drops/min
$11\frac{1}{4}$ drops/min $\Rightarrow$ 12 drops/min

EXAMPLE I   800 ml of fluid is to be given over 5 hours. The I.V. set delivers 15 drops/ml. At what rate should it drip?

$$\text{RATE (drops/min)} = \frac{\text{VOLUME (drops)}}{\text{TIME (minutes)}}$$

$$\therefore \text{RATE (drops/min)} = \frac{\text{VOLUME (drops)}}{\text{TIME (hours)} \times 60}$$

$$= \frac{800 \text{ ml} \times 15 \text{ drops/ml}}{5 \text{ hours} \times 60}$$

$$= \frac{800 \times 15}{5 \times 60} \text{ drops/min}$$

$$= 40 \text{ drops/min}$$

EXAMPLE 2   600 ml of fluid is dripping at 20 drops/min. The I.V. set delivers 15 drops/ml. How long will it take for the patient to receive the fluid?

$$\text{TIME (hours)} = \frac{\text{VOLUME (drops)}}{\text{RATE (drops/hour)}}$$

$$\therefore \text{TIME (hours)} = \frac{\text{VOLUME (drops)}}{\text{RATE (drops/min)} \times 60}$$

$$= \frac{600 \text{ ml} \times 15 \text{ drops/ml}}{20 \text{ drops/min} \times 60}$$

$$= \frac{600 \times 15}{20 \times 60} \text{ hours}$$

$$= 7\tfrac{1}{2} \text{ hours}$$

EXAMPLE 3   A 1 litre flask of normal saline is set up at 0600 hours running at 16 drops/min. After 10 hours the drip rate is increased to 24 drops/min. The drip chamber gives 15 drops/ml. By what time would the flask need to be replaced?

(a)   16 drop/min $= \dfrac{16}{15}$ ml/min (at 15 drops/ml)

$= \dfrac{16}{15} \times 60$ ml/h

$= 64$ ml/h

(b) 64 ml/h $\times$ 10 h $=$ 640 ml (delivered)

1 litre $=$ 1000 ml

1000 $-$ 640 $=$ 360 ml (remaining)

(C) TIME (hours) $= \dfrac{\text{VOLUME (drops)}}{\text{RATE (drops/hour)}}$

$= \dfrac{360 \text{ ml} \times 15 \text{ drops/ml}}{24 \text{ drops/min} \times 60}$

$= \dfrac{360 \times 15}{24 \times 60}$ hours

$= 3\frac{3}{4}$ h
$= 3$ h 45 min

(d) total running
       time $= 10$ h $+$ 3 h 45 min

$= 13$ h 45 min

$\therefore$ Replacement
       time $= 0600$ h $+$ 13 h 45 min

$= 1945$ hours

EXERCISE 5A

1. A patient is to have 800 ml of Hartmann's solution over 10 hours. The I.V. set delivers 15 drops per ml. Calculate the rate in drops per minute.

2. 50 ml of blood is to be given to a child over one hour. The drip chamber emits 60 drops per ml. Calculate the rate in drops per minute.

3. A boy is to receive 400 ml of dextrose 4% over 8 hours. The I.V. set emits 60 drops/ml. Calculate the rate in drops per minute.

4. 800 ml of fluid is to drip at 50 drops per minute. How long will the fluid last if the I.V. set delivers 15 drops/ml?

5. Half a litre of fluid is being given at 25 drops/min, 15 drops/ml. What time will it take to give this amount?

6. An I.V. set delivers 15 drops/ml. A patient is to receive one litre of dextrose 4% at 30 drops/min. How long will the infusion take?

EXERCISE 5B   Calculate the drip rate in drops per minute. The IV set delivers 60 drops/millilitre. If the answer is a mixed number, then use the *next whole number*.

1. A patient is to receive half a litre of dextrose 4% over ten hours.

2. An infant is ordered 150 ml of Hartmann's solution to run over 6 hours.

3. A child is to receive 250 ml of blood over 4 hours.

4. 0.9 litres of dextrose 4% in $\frac{1}{5}$ saline is to run over 24 hours.

5. 350 ml of dextrose 4% is to be given over 8 hours.

EXERCISE 5C   Calculate the drip rate in drops/min. The I.V. set emits 15 drops/ml. If the answer is a mixed number, then use the *next whole number*

1. An anaemic child must be given one unit of packed cells over 5 hours. One unit contains 500 ml.

2. A patient is to receive 1200 ml of Hartmann's solution over 16 hours.

3. An anaemic adult male is to be given 2 units of blood in 8 hours. One unit contains 500 ml.

4. Towards the end of a transfusion, a woman is still to be given $1\frac{1}{2}$ units of blood over 5 hours. One unit contains 500 ml.

5. A patient is to receive 800 ml of dextrose 4% over 12 hours.

6. A patient is to be given 900 ml of Hartmann's solution over 8 hours.

7. 300 ml of blood is to be transfused over 4 hours.

8. 600 ml of dextrose 4% and $\frac{1}{5}$ saline is to be given over 10 hours.

9. 75 ml of dextrose 4% is to run over 2 hours.

10. A patient is to receive half a litre of Hartmann's solution every 8 hours.

11. A patient is to be given 750 ml of dextrose 4% over 6 hours.

12. 1.4 litres of dextrose 4% and $\frac{1}{5}$ saline is to run over 10 hours.

13. One unit of packed red cells is to be run over 3 hours. One unit contains 500 ml.

14. A patient is to be given one unit of plasma over 6 hours. One unit contains 500 ml.

EXERCISE 5D   The drip chamber gives 15 drops/ml

1. A patient has two intravenous lines inserted. One is running at 45 ml/h; the other at 30 ml/h. What volume of fluid would this patient receive I.V. in a 24-hour period?

2. A patient is receiving fluid from *two* I.V. lines. The first line is running at a drip rate of 17 drops/min; the second line at 22 drops/min. Calculate the total volume of fluid that the patient would receive I.V. over 12 hours.

3. 850 ml of Hartmann's solution is to be given I.V. For the first 6 hours the solution is run at 85 ml/h then the rate is reduced to 40 ml/h. Find the total time taken to give the full volume.

4. 1200 ml of fluid is to be given I.V. The rate is set at 22 drops/min for 10 hours and then decreased to 16 drops/min until all the fluid has been given. Calculate the total time taken.

5. A patient is to receive 900 ml of dextrose 4% I.V. A flask is set up at 0800 hours running at 60 ml/h. After 5 hours the rate is increased to 75 ml/h. At what time will the I.V. be completed?

6. At 0400 hours, 1.1 litres of dextrose 4% and $\frac{1}{5}$ saline is set running at at 20 drops/min. After 7 hours the rate is reduced slightly to 18 drops/min. Calculate the finishing time.

7. A 1 litre I.V. flask of normal saline has been running since full for 5 hours at a rate of 20 drops/min. The doctor orders the remaining contents to be run through in the next 4 hours. Calculate the new drip rate.

8. A patient has been receiving part of 1 litre of fluid I.V. at a rate of 40 drops/min for 3 hours. A specialist then orders the rate slowed so that the remaining fluid will be run over the next 8 hours. Calculate the required drip rate.

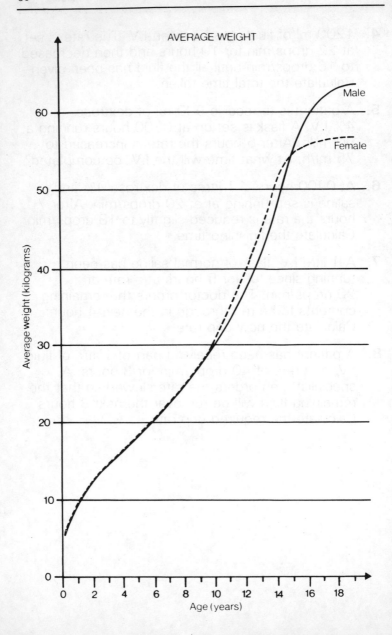

AVERAGE WEIGHT

Male

Female

Average weight (kilograms)

60

50

40

30

20

10

0

0   2   4   6   8   10   12   14   16   18

Age (years)

6. Paediatric dosages

Most drug dosages are based on the weight of a patient (although, for some groups of drugs, the dosages are based on body surface area).

The graph opposite shows the relationship between the age and average weight of males and females. Up until age 8, their average weights are nearly the same.

Great care must be taken when dispensing drugs for children as their range of weights is so wide. When dosages are prescribed in *micrograms*, write that unit *in full*, so as to avoid any confusion and prevent overdoses being given.

Overdoses can be fatal.

EXAMPLE 1   A child is prescribed erythromycin. The recommended dosage is 40 mg/kg/day, 4 doses daily. If the child's weight is 15 kg, calculate the size of a single dose.

$$
\begin{array}{r}
15 \text{ kg} \\
\times\ 40 \text{ mg/kg/day} \\
\hline
4\overline{)600} \text{ mg/day} \\
\hline
150 \text{ mg/dose}
\end{array}
$$

EXAMPLE 2   A child is to be given ampicillin. The recommended dosage is 80 mg/kg/day, 4 doses per day. Calculate the size of a single dose if the child's weight is 27 kg.

$$
\begin{array}{r}
27 \text{ kg} \\
\times\ 80 \text{ mg/kg/day} \\
\hline
4\overline{)2160} \text{ mg/day} \\
\hline
540 \text{ mg/dose}
\end{array}
$$

EXERCISE 6A   Calculate the size of a single dose
for a child weighing 12 kg:

1. Erythromycin, 40 mg/kg/day, 4 doses per day.
2. Penicillin V, 50 mg/kg/day, 4 doses per day.
3. Cephalexin, 30 mg/kg/day, 4 doses per day.

    Calculate the size of a single dose for a child
    weighing 20 kg:

4. Cloxacillin, 50 mg/kg/day, 4 doses per day.
5. Chloramphenicol, 60 mg/kg/day, 4 doses per day.
6. Ampicillin, 80 mg/kg/day, 4 doses per day.

    Calculate the size of a single dose for a child
    weighing 36 kg:

7. Methicillin, 100 mg/kg/day, 4 doses per day.
8. Streptomycin, 40 mg/kg/day, 3 doses per day.
9. Cephalothin (Keflin), 60 mg/kg/day, 4 doses per
    day.

EXAMPLE 3   A boy is ordered pethidine 35 mg, I.M., as premedication. Stock ampoules contain 50 mg in 1 ml. What volume must be withdrawn for injection?

$$\frac{\text{Volume}}{\text{required}} = \frac{\text{Strength required}}{\text{Stock strength}} \times \left(\begin{array}{c}\text{Volume of}\\\text{stock solution}\end{array}\right)$$

$$= \frac{35\,\text{mg}}{50\,\text{mg}} \times 1\,\text{ml}$$

$$= \frac{7}{10}\,\text{ml} \quad \text{or } 0{\cdot}7\,\text{ml}$$

EXAMPLE 4   An infant needs a maintenance injection of digoxin 40 micrograms. Paediatric ampoules contain 50 μg/2 ml. Calculate the amount to be drawn up.

$$\frac{\text{Volume}}{\text{required}} = \frac{\text{Strength required}}{\text{Stock strength}} \times \left(\begin{array}{c}\text{Volume of}\\\text{stock solution}\end{array}\right)$$

$$= \frac{40\,\text{micrograms}}{50\,\text{micrograms}} \times 2\,\text{ml}$$

$$= \frac{8}{5}\,\text{ml} \quad \text{or } 1{\cdot}6\,\text{ml}$$

EXAMPLE 5   A child with TB is to be given 125 mg of streptomycin by I.M.I. Stock on hand has a strength of 1 g in 2 ml. What volume of stock must be injected?

$$\frac{\text{Volume}}{\text{required}} = \frac{\text{Strength required}}{\text{Stock strength}} \times \left(\begin{array}{c}\text{Volume of}\\\text{stock solution}\end{array}\right)$$

$$= \frac{125\,\text{mg}}{1000\,\text{mg}} \times 2\,\text{ml}$$

$$= \frac{25}{100}\,\text{ml} \quad \text{or } 0{\cdot}25\,\text{ml}$$

EXERCISE 6B   Calculate the volume to be withdrawn for injection for each of these paediatric dosages:

	Ordered		Stock ampoule
1	Pethidine	20 mg	50 mg in 1 ml
2	Cortisone	10 mg	25 mg in 1 ml
3	Cortisone	20 mg	50 mg in 2 ml
4	Atropine	0·3 mg	0·4 mg in 1 ml
5	Digoxin	125 micrograms	0·5 mg/2 ml
6	Digoxin	18 micrograms	50 µg in 2 ml
7	Streptomycin	200 mg	1 gram in 2 ml
8	Streptomycin	150 mg	1 gram in 5 ml
9	Kanamycin	120 mg	500 mg in 2 ml
10	Kanamycin	300 mg	500 mg in 2 ml
11	Methicillin	400 mg	1 g in 3 ml
12	Sulphadimidine	100 mg	1 g in 3 ml
13	Phenobarb	50 mg	200 mg/ml
14	Phenobarb	120 mg	200 mg/ml
15	Morphine	6·5 mg	10 mg in 1 ml
16	Gentamicin	15 mg	20 mg/2 ml
17	Gentamicin	40 mg	60 mg/1·5 ml
18	Largactil	8 mg	10 mg/ml
19	Largactil	15 mg	25 mg/ml
20	Omnopon	16 mg	20 mg per ml

EXAMPLE 6 A child is ordered 80 mg of paracetamol elixir (Panadol). Stock on hand is 100 mg in 5 ml. Calculate the volume to be given.

$$\text{Volume required} = \frac{\text{Strength required}}{\text{Stock strength}} \times \left(\begin{array}{c}\text{Volume of}\\\text{stock solution}\end{array}\right)$$

$$= \frac{80\,\text{mg}}{100\,\text{mg}} \times 5\,\text{ml}$$

$$= 4\,\text{ml}$$

EXAMPLE 7 A child is to be given 175 micrograms of digoxin, orally. Paediatric mixture contains 50 micrograms per ml. Calculate the required volume.

$$\text{Volume required} = \frac{\text{Strength required}}{\text{Stock strength}} \times \left(\begin{array}{c}\text{Volume of}\\\text{stock solution}\end{array}\right)$$

$$= \frac{175\,\text{micrograms}}{50\,\text{micrograms}} \times 1\,\text{ml}$$

$$= \frac{7}{2}\,\text{ml} \quad \text{or } 3 \cdot 5\,\text{ml}$$

EXAMPLE 8 A child is prescribed 180 mg of aspirin. On hand is a mixture containing 150 mg in 5 ml. How much should be given?

$$\text{Volume required} = \frac{\text{Strength required}}{\text{Stock strength}} \times \left(\begin{array}{c}\text{Volume of}\\\text{stock solution}\end{array}\right)$$

$$= \frac{180\,\text{mg}}{150\,\text{mg}} \times 5\,\text{ml}$$

$$= 6\,\text{ml}$$

EXERCISE 6C   Calculate the volume to be given orally for these paediatric dosages. (The strength of the stock mixture is given in brackets.)

1. 70 mg of paracetamol elixir
   (100 mg/5 ml)

2. 300 mg of Panadol
   (120 mg/5 ml)

3. 600 mg of sulphadimidine
   (500 mg/5 ml)

4. 900 mg of sulphadimidine
   (500 mg/5 ml)

5. 125 micrograms of digoxin
   (50 micrograms/ml)

6. 200 mg of penicillin
   (125 mg/5 ml)

7. 350 mg of penicillin
   (125 mg/5 ml)

8. 15 mg of Largactil
   (25 mg/5 ml)

9. 120 mg of aspirin
   (150 mg/5 ml)

10. 200 mg of aspirin
    (150 mg/5 ml)

7. Summary exercises

SUMMARY EXERCISE I

1. A patient is ordered erythromycin 135 mg, I.M.I. Stock vials contain 300 mg/10 ml. Calculate the volume required for injection.

2. 300 000 units of Bicillin are to be given by I.M.I On hand is Bicillin 1.2 megaunits in 2 ml. What volume should be drawn up?

3. 375 mg of penicillin is required. Stock on hand is 250 mg tablets. How many tablets should be given?

4. A patient is ordered 360 mg of Pensig, orally. The strength of the stock syrup is 125 mg/5 ml. Calculate the volume required.

5. A solution has a strength of $12\frac{1}{2}\%$. Express $12\frac{1}{2}\%$ as a *ratio* strength.

6. 5 litres of normal saline solution (0.9%) is to be prepared. What volume of (a) stock 18% saline (b) water must be used?

7. Calculate the amount of (a) stock solution (b) distilled water, to make $2\frac{1}{2}$ litres of lotion, strength 1 in 50, from stock lotion of strength 1 in 10.

8. 1.2 litres of thymol 1 in 8 is to be prepared.
   (a) What quantity of *pure* stock is required?
   (b) How much water must be added?

9. How many grams of sodium bicarbonate should be used to prepare 2 litres of a $2\frac{1}{2}$% solution?

10. 700 ml of Hartmann's solution is to be given over 8 hours. The I.V. set delivers 15 drops/ml. At what rate should it drip?

11. 800 ml of fluid is to be given I.V. The fluid is run at 70 ml/h for the first 5 hours then the rate is reduced to 60 ml/h.
Find the total time taken to give the 800 ml.

12. A child is prescribed penicillin V. The recommended dosage is 50 mg/kg/day; 4 doses daily. If the child's weight is 18 kg, calculate the size of a single dose.

13. A girl is ordered phenobarb 140 mg. Stock ampoules contain 200 mg/ml.
What volume must be withdrawn for injection?

14. A child is prescribed 175 mg streptomycin by I.M.I. A stock ampoule contains 1 g in 2 ml. What volume of stock must be injected?

15. A young boy is to have 125 micrograms of digoxin, orally. Paediatric mixture has a strength of 50 micrograms per ml. Calculate the required volume.

SUMMARY EXERCISE II

1. An injection of digoxin 225 micrograms is
    ordered. Stock on hand is digoxin 500
    micrograms in 2 ml. What volume of stock should
    be given?

2. How many 30 mg tablets of phenobarb should be
    given if phenobarb 15 mg is prescribed?

3. 900 mg of penicillin is to be given orally. Stock
    mixture contains 250 mg/5ml. Calculate the
    volume of mixture to be given.

4. Calculate the percentage strength when 5 ml of
    disinfectant concentrate is mixed with water to
    make 1 litre of solution.

5. Calculate the percentage strength of the solution
    made by dissolving 20 g of dextrose in 500 ml
    of water.

6. A nebulizer is to be used to give 4 ml of 0.2%
    salbutamol. Stock solution has a strength of 0.5%
    salbutamol. Calculate the required volume of
    (a) stock (b) water.

7. Calculate the amount of (a) stock solution
    (b) distilled water to make 800 ml of chlorhexidine
    1:2000 from 2% stock solution.

8. What volume of pure Savlon is needed to prepare
    2.4 litres of a 5% solution? How much water
    must be added?

9. Calculate the volume of 4% dextrose which
    contains 70 g of dextrose.

10. 750 ml of dextrose 4% is dripping at 30 drops/min.
The I.V. set delivers 15 drops/ml.
How long will it take for the patient to receive this fluid?

11. A patient is to be given 1.2 litres of fluid I.V. The rate is set initially at 15 drops/min and then after 12 hours is increased to 24 drops/min. Calculate the total running time.

12. A child is to be given streptomycin.
The recommended dosage is 40 mg/kg/day;
3 doses per day. Calculate the size of a single dose if the child's weight is 24 kg.

13. It is necessary to give an infant an injection of digoxin 35 micrograms.
Paediatric ampoules contain 50 µg/2 ml.
Calculate the amount to be drawn up.

14. A boy is ordered 120 mg of paracetamol elixir.
Stock on hand has a strength of 100 mg/5 ml.
What volume should be given?

15. A young girl is prescribed 700 mg of sulphadimidine, to be taken orally. The stock mixture contains 500 mg/5 ml. How much mixture should be given?

Answers to diagnostic test

		Reference (*EXERCISE*)
1.	**(a)** 830 **(b)** 8300 **(c)** 83 000	1A
2.	**(a)** 0·258 **(b)** 2·58 **(c)** 25·8	1A
3.	**(a)** 0·378 **(b)** 0·0378 **(c)** 0·003 78	1B
4.	**(a)** 56·9 **(b)** 5·69 **(c)** 0·569	1B
5.	**(a)** 1000 **(b)** 1000 **(c)** 1000	1C
6.	**(a)** 780 mg **(b)** 0·034 grams	1C
7.	**(a)** 86 micrograms **(b)** 0·294 mg	1C
8.	**(a)** 2400 ml **(b)** 0·965 litres	1C
9.	**(a)** 27 **(b)** 2·7 **(c)** 0·27 **(d)** 0·0027	1D
10.	**(a)** 468 **(b)** 4·68 **(c)** 4·68 **(d)** 0·468	1D
11.	675 ml	1E
12.	2150 ml or 2·15 litres	1E
13.	2, 3, 6, 7 and 9 are factors	1F
14.	**(a)** $\frac{2}{3}$ **(b)** $\frac{7}{9}$	1G
15.	**(a)** $\frac{3}{40}$ **(b)** $\frac{7}{16}$	1G
16.	**(a)** $\frac{4}{5}$ **(b)** $\frac{2}{3}$ **(c)** $\frac{3}{5}$	1H
17.	**(a)** $\frac{7}{10}$ **(b)** $\frac{4}{5}$ **(c)** $\frac{2}{5}$	1H
18.	**(a)** 0·9 **(b)** 0·6 **(c)** 0·5	1I
19.	**(a)** 0·2 **(b)** 0·4 **(c)** 0·8	1I
20.	**(a)** 0·625 **(b)** 0·45 **(c)** 0·68 **(d)** 0·775	1J

	Reference (*EXERCISE*)
21. (a) 0·71 (b) 0·78	1J
22. (a) 0·233 (b) 0·843	1J
23. (a) 75% (b) 65% (c) 32%	1K
24. (a) $33\frac{1}{3}$% (b) $62\frac{1}{2}$% (c) $55\frac{5}{9}$%	1K
25. (a) 1 in 5 (b) 1 in 21	1L
26. (a) 1:3 (b) 1:29	1L
27. 200 ml	1L
28. 80 ml	1L
29. (a) 20% (b) 2% (c) 0·2% (d) 0·02%	1M
30. (a) $\frac{3}{10}$ (b) $\frac{6}{10} = \frac{3}{5}$ (c) $\frac{8}{10} = \frac{4}{5}$	1N
31. (a) $\frac{55}{100} = \frac{11}{20}$ (b) $\frac{72}{100} = \frac{18}{25}$ (c) $\frac{68}{100} = \frac{17}{25}$ (d) $\frac{9}{100}$	1N
32. (a) $\frac{6}{100} = \frac{3}{50}$ (b) $\frac{43}{100}$ (c) $\frac{75}{100} = \frac{3}{4}$	1O
33. (a) $\frac{7}{1000}$ (b) $\frac{3}{10000}$ (c) $\frac{5}{10000} = \frac{1}{2000}$	1O
34. (a) $\frac{1}{200}$ (b) $\frac{11}{200}$ (c) $\frac{35}{200} = \frac{7}{40}$	1O
35. (a) $\frac{5}{9}$ (b) $1\frac{1}{14}$ (c) $\frac{2}{5}$	1P
36. (a) $1\frac{2}{3}$ (b) $\frac{5}{7}$ (c) $\frac{25}{28}$	1Q
37. (a) 117 cm (b) 135 cm (c) 173 cm	1R
38. (a) 47 kg (b) 68 kg (c) 86 kg	1S

Answers

Chapter 1 : A review of basic calculations

EXERCISE 1A

MULTIPLICATION BY 10, 100, 1000

(1) 6·8, 68, 680

(2) 9·75, 97·5, 975

(3) 37, 370, 3700

(4) 56·2, 562, 5620

(5) 770, 7700, 77 000

(6) 8250, 82 500, 825 000

(7) 2, 20, 200

(8) 0·46, 4·6, 46

(9) 0·147, 1·47, 14·7

(10) 0·06, 0·6, 6

(11) 37·6, 376, 3760

(12) 6·39, 63·9, 639

(13) 0·75, 7·5, 75

(14) 0·8, 8, 80

(15) 0·03, 0·3, 3

(16) 0·505, 5·05, 50·5

EXERCISE 1B

DIVISION BY 10, 100, 1000

(1) 9·84, 0·984, 0·0984

(2) 0·591, 0·0591, 0·005 91

(3) 0·26, 0·026, 0·0026

(4) 30·7, 3·07, 0·307

(5) 8·2, 0·82, 0·082

(6) 0·7, 0·07, 0·007

(7) 0·3, 0·03, 0·003

(8) 0·75, 0·075, 0·0075

(9) 6·8, 0·68, 0·068

(10) 0·229, 0·0229, 0·002 29

(11) 5.14, 0.514, 0·0514

(12) 91·6, 9·16, 0·916

(13) 6·72, 0·672, 0·0672

(14) 38·7, 3·87, 0·387

(15) 0·894, 0·0894, 0·008 94

(16) 0·0707, 0·007 07, 0·000 707

EXERCISE 1C

CONVERTING METRIC UNITS

Milligrams:

(1) 4000   **(2)** 8700   **(3)** 690   **(4)** 20

(5) 35   **(6)** 6   **(7)** 655   **(8)** 4280

Grams:

(9) 6   **(10)** 7·25   **(11)** 0·865   **(12)** 0·095

(13) 0·07   **(14)** 0·002   **(15)** 0·005   **(16)** 0·125

Micrograms:

(17)	195	**(18)**	600	**(19)**	750	**(20)**	75
(21)	80	**(22)**	1	**(23)**	625	**(24)**	98

Milligrams:

(25)	0·825	**(26)**	0·75	**(27)**	0·065	**(28)**	0·095
(29)	0·01	**(30)**	0·005	**(31)**	0·2	**(32)**	0·03

Millilitres:

(33)	2000	**(34)**	30 000	**(35)**	1500	**(36)**	4500
(37)	1600	**(38)**	2240	**(39)**	800	**(40)**	750

Litres:

(41)	4	**(42)**	10	**(43)**	0·625	**(44)**	0·35
(45)	0·095	**(46)**	0·06	**(47)**	0·005	**(48)**	0·002

EXERCISE 1D

MULTIPLICATION OF DECIMALS

- **(1)** 45, 4·5, 0·45, 0·45
- **(2)** 14, 0·14, 0·014, 0·0014
- **(3)** 12, 0·12, 0·12, 0·0012
- **(4)** 36, 0·36, 0·0036, 0·0036
- **(5)** 56, 5·6, 0·56, 0·0056
- **(6)** 102, 10·2, 1·02, 0·102
- **(7)** 152, 15·2, 0·152, 0·152
- **(8)** 46, 0·46, 0·046, 0·0046
- **(9)** 145, 1·45, 1·45, 1·45
- **(10)** 93, 0·93, 0·0093, 0·093
- **(11)** 333, 33·3, 0·333, 0·0333
- **(12)** 287, 0·287, 0·0287, 2·87
- **(13)** 192, 0·0192, 0·192, 0·0192
- **(14)** 616, 6·16, 0·0616, 0·616
- **(15)** 768, 0·768, 0·0768, 0·0768

EXERCISE 1E

DILUTING SOLUTIONS

Answers in millilitres (ml) :

(1) 500	**(2)** 450	**(3)** 525
(4) 500	**(5)** 625	**(6)** 475
(7) 800	**(8)** 850	**(9)** 915
(10) 950	**(11)** 1035	**(12)** 825
(13) 820	**(14)** 775	**(15)** 955
(16) 1650	**(17)** 1575	**(18)** 1785
(19) 1350	**(20)** 1325	**(21)** 1265
(22) 2700	**(23)** 2850	**(24)** 3305
(25) 2850	**(26)** 2725	**(27)** 2965
(28) 4350	**(29)** 3990	**(30)** 3875

EXERCISE 1F

FACTORS

(1) 2, 4, 5	**(11)** 4, 9, 12, 18
(2) 3, 4, 12	**(12)** 3, 5, 12, 15
(3) 3, 5, 15	**(13)** 3, 5, 9, 15
(4) 2, 8, 14	**(14)** 4, 8, 12, 16, 18, 24
(5) 3, 4, 12, 15, 20	**(15)** 5, 15, 25
(6) 3, 4, 6, 12, 18	**(16)** 3, 5, 11, 15
(7) 3, 5, 15, 25	**(17)** 5, 7
(8) 5, 17	**(18)** 4, 12, 15
(9) 3, 8, 12, 16, 24	**(19)** 4, 6, 8, 12, 16
(10) 5, 20, 25	**(20)** 6, 14, 15.

EXERCISE 1G

SIMPLIFYING FRACTIONS 1

Part a

(1) $\frac{2}{3}$	**(6)** $\frac{5}{7}$	**(11)** $\frac{7}{8}$	**(16)** $\frac{1}{3}$	**(21)** $\frac{9}{14}$
(2) $\frac{5}{7}$	**(7)** $\frac{5}{6}$	**(12)** $\frac{2}{3}$	**(17)** $\frac{2}{3}$	**(22)** $\frac{4}{5}$
(3) $\frac{3}{8}$	**(8)** $\frac{4}{5}$	**(13)** $\frac{3}{7}$	**(18)** $\frac{7}{8}$	**(23)** $\frac{13}{16}$
(4) $\frac{1}{2}$	**(9)** $\frac{3}{7}$	**(14)** $\frac{8}{9}$	**(19)** $\frac{18}{25}$	**(24)** $\frac{3}{10}$
(5) $\frac{3}{4}$	**(10)** $\frac{3}{10}$	**(15)** $\frac{2}{5}$	**(20)** $\frac{5}{11}$	**(25)** $\frac{4}{9}$

Part b

(1) $\frac{1}{2}$	**(5)** $\frac{1}{2}$	**(9)** $\frac{2}{15}$	**(13)** $\frac{5}{8}$	**(17)** $\frac{7}{9}$
(2) $\frac{3}{8}$	**(6)** $\frac{5}{12}$	**(10)** $\frac{8}{35}$	**(14)** $\frac{3}{4}$	**(18)** $\frac{3}{4}$
(3) $\frac{3}{10}$	**(7)** $\frac{5}{16}$	**(11)** $\frac{3}{10}$	**(15)** $\frac{11}{16}$	**(19)** $\frac{17}{24}$
(4) $\frac{1}{4}$	**(8)** $\frac{1}{4}$	**(12)** $\frac{4}{25}$	**(16)** $\frac{4}{9}$	**(20)** $\frac{13}{30}$

EXERCISE 1H

SIMPLIFYING FRACTIONS 2

(1) $\frac{3}{5}$	**(7)** $\frac{13}{15}$	**(13)** $\frac{2}{3}$	**(19)** $\frac{2}{3}$	**(25)** $\frac{2}{3}$	**(31)** $\frac{5}{6}$
(2) $\frac{2}{3}$	**(8)** $\frac{2}{3}$	**(14)** $\frac{2}{5}$	**(20)** $\frac{3}{4}$	**(26)** $\frac{8}{15}$	**(32)** $\frac{1}{6}$
(3) $\frac{3}{4}$	**(9)** $\frac{2}{5}$	**(15)** $\frac{9}{10}$	**(21)** $\frac{9}{10}$	**(27)** $\frac{5}{6}$	**(33)** $\frac{3}{20}$
(4) $\frac{5}{12}$	**(10)** $\frac{3}{4}$	**(16)** $\frac{3}{5}$	**(22)** $\frac{3}{4}$	**(28)** $\frac{14}{25}$	**(34)** $\frac{3}{8}$
(5) $\frac{2}{3}$	**(11)** $\frac{5}{8}$	**(17)** $\frac{9}{10}$	**(23)** $\frac{15}{16}$	**(29)** $\frac{4}{5}$	**(35)** $\frac{3}{10}$
(6) $\frac{5}{6}$	**(12)** $\frac{3}{8}$	**(18)** $\frac{6}{25}$	**(24)** $\frac{2}{5}$	**(30)** $\frac{7}{10}$	**(36)** $\frac{11}{16}$

EXERCISE 1I

CONVERTING VULGAR FRACTIONS TO TENTHS

Part a

(1) $0.3 = \frac{3}{10}$	**(6)** $0.2 = \frac{2}{10}$	**(11)** $0.8 = \frac{8}{10}$	**(16)** $1.0 = \frac{10}{10}$
(2) $0.6 = \frac{6}{10}$	**(7)** $0.7 = \frac{7}{10}$	**(12)** $0.1 = \frac{1}{10}$	**(17)** $0.7 = \frac{7}{10}$
(3) $0.9 = \frac{9}{10}$	**(8)** $0.2 = \frac{2}{10}$	**(13)** $0.5 = \frac{5}{10}$	**(18)** $0.5 = \frac{5}{10}$
(4) $0.4 = \frac{4}{10}$	**(9)** $0.7 = \frac{7}{10}$	**(14)** $0.2 = \frac{2}{10}$	**(19)** $0.4 = \frac{4}{10}$
(5) $0.8 = \frac{8}{10}$	**(10)** $0.5 = \frac{5}{10}$	**(15)** $0.5 = \frac{5}{10}$	**(20)** $0.8 = \frac{8}{10}$

Part b

(1) $0.5 = \frac{5}{10}$	**(7)** $0.8 = \frac{8}{10}$	**(13)** $0.7 = \frac{7}{10}$	**(19)** $0.1 = \frac{1}{10}$
(2) $0.3 = \frac{3}{10}$	**(8)** $0.2 = \frac{2}{10}$	**(14)** $0.9 = \frac{9}{10}$	**(20)** $0.2 = \frac{2}{10}$
(3) $0.7 = \frac{7}{10}$	**(9)** $0.8 = \frac{8}{10}$	**(15)** $0.1 = \frac{1}{10}$	**(21)** $0.4 = \frac{4}{10}$
(4) $0.2 = \frac{2}{10}$	**(10)** $0.1 = \frac{1}{10}$	**(16)** $0.4 = \frac{4}{10}$	**(22)** $0.6 = \frac{6}{10}$
(5) $0.4 = \frac{4}{10}$	**(11)** $0.3 = \frac{3}{10}$	**(17)** $0.6 = \frac{6}{10}$	**(23)** $0.8 = \frac{8}{10}$
(6) $0.6 = \frac{6}{10}$	**(12)** $0.4 = \frac{4}{10}$	**(18)** $0.9 = \frac{9}{10}$	**(24)** $0.9 = \frac{9}{10}$

EXERCISE 1J

VULGAR FRACTION TO A DECIMAL

Part a

(1) 0.5	**(6)** 0.125	**(11)** 0.04	**(16)** 0.275
(2) 0.25	**(7)** 0.875	**(12)** 0.28	**(17)** 0.675
(3) 0.75	**(8)** 0.05	**(13)** 0.88	**(18)** 0.02
(4) 0.4	**(9)** 0.35	**(14)** 0.025	**(19)** 0.0125
(5) 0.6	**(10)** 0.65	**(15)** 0.225	**(20)** 0.2375

Part b

(1) 0.33	**(6)** 0.43	**(11)** 0.033	**(16)** 0.283
(2) 0.67	**(7)** 0.86	**(12)** 0.367	**(17)** 0.014
(3) 0.17	**(8)** 0.11	**(13)** 0.967	**(18)** 0.129
(4) 0.83	**(9)** 0.56	**(14)** 0.017	**(19)** 0.011
(5) 0.14	**(10)** 0.89	**(15)** 0.117	**(20)** 0.522

EXERCISE 1K
VULGAR FRACTION TO A PERCENTAGE

(1) 50%	**(11)** 90%	**(21)** 28%	**(31)** $87\frac{1}{2}$%
(2) 25%	**(12)** 5%	**(22)** 44%	**(32)** $16\frac{2}{3}$%
(3) 75%	**(13)** 15%	**(23)** 52%	**(33)** $83\frac{1}{3}$%
(4) 20%	**(14)** 45%	**(24)** 68%	**(34)** $11\frac{1}{9}$%
(5) 40%	**(15)** 55%	**(25)** 76%	**(35)** $44\frac{4}{9}$%
(6) 60%	**(16)** 65%	**(26)** 92%	**(36)** $77\frac{7}{9}$%
(7) 80%	**(17)** 85%	**(27)** $33\frac{1}{3}$%	**(37)** $2\frac{1}{2}$%
(8) 10%	**(28)** 95%	**(28)** $66\frac{2}{3}$%	**(38)** $7\frac{1}{2}$%
(9) 30%	**(19)** 4%	**(29)** $12\frac{1}{2}$%	**(39)** $22\frac{1}{2}$%
(10) 70%	**(20)** 12%	**(30)** $62\frac{1}{2}$%	**(40)** $27\frac{1}{2}$%

EXERCISE 1L
DILUTION RATIOS
Part a

(1) 1 in 3	**(4)** 1 in 11	**(7)** 1 in 31	**(10)** 1 in 201
(2) 1 in 6	**(5)** 1 in 16	**(8)** 1 in 51	**(11)** 1 in 251
(3) 1 in 8	**(6)** 1 in 26	**(9)** 1 in 101	**(12)** 1 in 501

Part b

(1) 1:1	**(4)** 1:6	**(7)** 1:19	**(10)** 1:49
(2) 1:2	**(5)** 1:9	**(8)** 1:24	**(11)** 1:99
(3) 1:4	**(6)** 1:14	**(9)** 1:39	**(12)** 1:199

Part c (millilitres)

(1) 25,20	**(5)** 70, 60	**(9)** 150, 129
(2) 75, 50	**(6)** 55, 50	**(10)** 143, 125
(3) 60, 50	**(7)** 133, 100	**(11)** 250, 222
(4) 200, 150	**(8)** 188, 150	**(12)** 556, 500

EXERCISE 1M

RATIO TO PERCENTAGE

(1)	50%	**(17)**	33·33%	**(33)**	0·13%
(2)	25%	**(18)**	16·67%	**(34)**	0·11%
(3)	20%	**(19)**	14·29%	**(35)**	Relationships:
(4)	10%	**(20)**	12·5%		1 in 20 = $\frac{1}{10}$ of 1 in 2
(5)	5%	**(21)**	11·11%		1 in 200 = $\frac{1}{10}$ of 1 in 20
(6)	4%	**(22)**	8·33%		1 in 30 = $\frac{1}{10}$ of 1 in 3
(7)	2%	**(23)**	6·67%		1 in 300 = $\frac{1}{10}$ of 1 in 30
(8)	1%	**(24)**	3·33%	**(36)**	33·33%
(9)	0·5%	**(25)**	1·67%	**(37)**	25%
(10)	0·4%	**(26)**	1·43%	**(38)**	16·67%
(11)	0·25%	**(27)**	1·33%	**(39)**	14·29%
(12)	0·1%	**(28)**	1·25%	**(40)**	12·5%
(13)	0·05%	**(29)**	1·11%	**(41)**	11·11%
(14)	0·04%	**(30)**	0·33%	**(42)**	10%
(15)	0·02%	**(31)**	0·25%		
(16)	0·01%	**(32)**	0·14%		

EXERCISE 1N

DECIMAL FRACTION TO VULGAR FRACTION

Part a

(1)	$\frac{1}{10}$	**(3)**	$\frac{3}{10}$	**(5)**	$\frac{3}{5}$	**(7)**	$\frac{4}{5}$
(2)	$\frac{1}{5}$	**(4)**	$\frac{1}{2}$	**(6)**	$\frac{7}{10}$	**(8)**	$\frac{9}{10}$

Part b

(1)	$\frac{6}{25}$	**(11)**	$\frac{3}{100}$	**(21)**	$\frac{3}{4}$	**(31)**	$\frac{57}{100}$
(2)	$\frac{23}{50}$	**(12)**	$\frac{18}{25}$	**(22)**	$\frac{13}{50}$	**(32)**	$\frac{87}{100}$
(3)	$\frac{77}{100}$	**(13)**	$\frac{13}{20}$	**(23)**	$\frac{39}{100}$	**(33)**	$\frac{41}{100}$
(4)	$\frac{13}{100}$	**(14)**	$\frac{1}{4}$	**(24)**	$\frac{53}{100}$	**(34)**	$\frac{2}{25}$
(5)	$\frac{7}{20}$	**(15)**	$\frac{9}{25}$	**(25)**	$\frac{9}{50}$	**(35)**	$\frac{16}{25}$
(6)	$\frac{81}{100}$	**(16)**	$\frac{29}{50}$	**(26)**	$\frac{69}{100}$	**(36)**	$\frac{7}{25}$
(7)	$\frac{33}{50}$	**(17)**	$\frac{4}{25}$	**(27)**	$\frac{12}{25}$	**(37)**	$\frac{79}{100}$
(8)	$\frac{1}{100}$	**(18)**	$\frac{83}{100}$	**(28)**	$\frac{1}{20}$	**(38)**	$\frac{19}{50}$
(9)	$\frac{19}{20}$	**(19)**	$\frac{9}{20}$	**(29)**	$\frac{17}{20}$	**(39)**	$\frac{99}{100}$
(10)	$\frac{11}{20}$	**(20)**	$\frac{24}{25}$	**(30)**	$\frac{23}{25}$	**(40)**	$\frac{3}{20}$

EXERCISE 1O

PERCENTAGE TO VULGAR FRACTION

Part a

(1) $\frac{1}{50}$ (4) $\frac{1}{20}$ (7) $\frac{3}{25}$ (10) $\frac{3}{10}$ (13) $\frac{9}{20}$
(2) $\frac{3}{100}$ (5) $\frac{7}{100}$ (8) $\frac{3}{20}$ (11) $\frac{7}{20}$ (14) $\frac{1}{2}$
(3) $\frac{1}{25}$ (6) $\frac{1}{10}$ (9) $\frac{1}{5}$ (12) $\frac{2}{5}$ (15) $\frac{9}{10}$

Part b

(1) $\frac{1}{1000}$ (6) $\frac{7}{1000}$ (11) $\frac{1}{2500}$
(2) $\frac{1}{500}$ (7) $\frac{1}{125}$ (12) $\frac{1}{2000}$
(3) $\frac{1}{250}$ (8) $\frac{9}{1000}$ (13) $\frac{3}{5000}$
(4) $\frac{1}{200}$ (9) $\frac{1}{10000}$ (14) $\frac{7}{10000}$
(5) $\frac{3}{500}$ (10) $\frac{1}{5000}$ (15) $\frac{9}{10000}$

Part c

(1) $\frac{1}{200}$ (3) $\frac{1}{40}$ (5) $\frac{3}{40}$
(2) $\frac{3}{200}$ (4) $\frac{9}{200}$ (6) $\frac{1}{8}$

EXERCISE 1P

MULTIPLICATION OF VULGAR FRACTIONS

(1) $\frac{1}{5}$ (10) $\frac{3}{20}$ (19) $\frac{9}{10}$ (28) $\frac{3}{16}$
(2) $\frac{5}{24}$ (11) $\frac{4}{9}$ (20) $\frac{9}{32}$ (29) $\frac{2}{15}$
(3) $\frac{5}{9}$ (12) $\frac{1}{18}$ (21) 1   (30) $\frac{1}{5}$
(4) $\frac{1}{6}$ (13) $\frac{11}{42}$ (22) $\frac{1}{135}$ (31) $\frac{27}{32}$
(5) $1\frac{2}{3}$ (14) $\frac{3}{140}$ (23) $\frac{7}{18}$ (32) $\frac{1}{18}$
(6) $\frac{3}{50}$ (15) $\frac{20}{21}$ (24) $\frac{5}{27}$ (33) $\frac{1}{360}$
(7) $\frac{3}{5}$ (16) $\frac{12}{35}$ (25) $\frac{7}{15}$ (34) $\frac{7}{72}$
(8) $\frac{9}{20}$ (17) $\frac{5}{28}$ (26) $\frac{7}{16}$ (35) $\frac{21}{160}$
(9) $\frac{5}{6}$ (18) $\frac{1}{16}$ (27) $\frac{4}{27}$ (36) $\frac{121}{160}$

EXERCISE 1Q

DIVISION BY A VULGAR FRACTION

(1) $\frac{2}{3}$	**(10)** $3\frac{3}{4}$	**(19)** $\frac{10}{21}$	**(28)** $\frac{1}{3}$
(2) $1\frac{1}{2}$	**(11)** $\frac{3}{5}$	**(20)** $1\frac{5}{7}$	**(29)** $2\frac{2}{3}$
(3) $1\frac{1}{3}$	**(12)** $\frac{2}{3}$	**(21)** $\frac{3}{14}$	**(30)** $\frac{8}{9}$
(4) $\frac{3}{5}$	**(13)** $\frac{2}{3}$	**(22)** $1\frac{1}{7}$	**(31)** $1\frac{1}{9}$
(5) 4	**(14)** $1\frac{1}{5}$	**(23)** $\frac{1}{7}$	**(32)** $1\frac{1}{3}$
(6) $1\frac{1}{2}$	**(15)** $\frac{3}{14}$	**(24)** $\frac{5}{12}$	**(33)** $\frac{7}{10}$
(7) $\frac{1}{2}$	**(16)** $2\frac{1}{12}$	**(25)** $\frac{3}{4}$	**(34)** $\frac{9}{25}$
(8) $\frac{5}{16}$	**(17)** $1\frac{1}{7}$	**(26)** $1\frac{3}{4}$	**(35)** $\frac{4}{5}$
(9) $\frac{9}{10}$	**(18)** $\frac{5}{14}$	**(27)** $\frac{5}{9}$	**(36)** $1\frac{1}{2}$

EXERCISE 1R

CONVERTING UNITS OF LENGTH

To the nearest cm:

(1) 81	**(4)** 102	**(7)** 147	**(10)** 175	**(13)** 196
(2) 89	**(5)** 119	**(8)** 137	**(11)** 158	**(14)** 203
(3) 109	**(6)** 130	**(9)** 165	**(12)** 185	**(15)** 219

EXERCISE 1S

CONVERTING UNITS OF WEIGHT

To the nearest kilogram:

(1) 24	**(4)** 40	**(7)** 58	**(10)** 77	**(13)** 98	**(16)** 118
(2) 27	**(5)** 50	**(8)** 69	**(11)** 84	**(14)** 105	**(17)** 125
(3) 37	**(6)** 55	**(9)** 72	**(12)** 92	**(15)** 112	**(18)** 128

Chapter 2: Drug dosages for injection

All answers are in millilitres (ml)

EXERCISE 2A

(1) 0·8	**(2)** 1·4	**(3)** 6·4	**(4)** 4
(5) 1·3	**(6)** 1·7	**(7)** 1·5	

EXERCISE 2B

(1) 1·5	**(2)** 3·2	**(3)** 0·6	**(4)** 4
(5) 0·8	**(6)** 0·2	**(7)** 1·3	

EXERCISE 2C

(1) 1·6	**(2)** 1·2	**(3)** 1·2	**(4)** 0·25
(5) 2·4	**(6)** 3	**(7)** 0·6	**(8)** 0·6
(9) 0·8			

EXERCISE 2D
    (1) 6·7   **(2)** 1·3   **(3)** 0·83   **(4)** 0·67
    (5) 0·67   **(6)** 0·43   **(7)** 7·2   **(8)** 1·8
    (9) 1·3

EXERCISE 2E
    (1) 0·6   **(2)** 0·28   **(3)** 7   **(4)** 0·6
    (5) 0·35   **(6)** 1·6   **(7)** 1·2   **(8)** 0·8
    (9) 3   **(10)** 3·6   **(11)** 4   **(12)** 0·3
   (13) 1·5   **(14)** 7·5   **(15)** 0·75   **(16)** 6·3
   (17) 1·7   **(18)** 0·75   **(19)** 1·5   **(20)** 0·72

Chapter 3: Dosages of tablets and mixtures

EXERCISE 3A   Number of tablets
    (1) 3   **(2)** 2   **(3)** $1\frac{1}{2}$ **(4)** $\frac{1}{2}$
    (5) $2\frac{1}{2}$ **(6)** $\frac{1}{4}$ **(7)** $1\frac{1}{2}$

EXERCISE 3B   Volume in ml
    (1) 20   **(2)** 15   **(3)** 30   **(4)** 20   **(5)** 25
    (6) 30   **(7)** 20   **(8)** 7   **(9)** 24   **(10)** 32

Chapter 4: Dilution and strengths of solutions

EXERCISE 4A
    (1) a. 1 in 1000 **b.** 1 in 100 **c.** 1 in 10
    (2) a. 1 in 2 **b.** 1 in 4 **c.** 1 in 5 **d.** 1 in 10 **e.** 1 in 20 **f.** 1 in 40 **g.** 1 in 50 **h.** 1 in 200 **i.** 1 in 500 **j.** 1 in 1000
    (3) a. 1 in 25 **b.** 4%
    (4) a. 1 in 20 **b.** 5%
    (5) $1\frac{1}{4}\% = 1·25\%$
    (6) a. 0·05% **b.** 0·02%
    (7) $2\frac{1}{2}\%$

EXERCISE 4B   All answers in ml
    (1) a. 50, 950 **b.** 100, 1900 **c.** 60, 1140
    (2) a. 100, 400 **b.** 150, 600 **c.** 500, 2000
    (3) 5, 195 **(4)** 12·5, 487·5
    (5) 15, 15 **(6)** 100, 100 **(7)** 2·4, 1·6
    (8) 3·6, 2·4 **(9)** 50, 450 **(10)** 250, 750

EXERCISE 4C   All answers in ml
- **(1)** 200, 800   **(2)** 250, 1250   **(3)** 250, 250
- **(4)** 750, 750   **(5)** 120, 480   **(6)** 600, 2400 ·
- **(7)** 125, 2375   **(8)** 40, 1960   **(9)** 7, 693
- **(10)** 400, 400

EXERCISE 4D   All answers in ml
- **(1)** 40, 760   **(2)** 150, 1350   **(3)** 50, 4950
- **(4)** 250, 2250   **(5)** 50, 950   **(6)** 30, 1170
- **(7)** 3·5, 346·5   **(8)** 125, 875   **(9)** 37·5, 262·5
- **(10)** 6·25, 93·75

EXERCISE 4E
- **(1)** 100 mg
- **(2)** 50 mg
- **(3) a.** 30 g **b.** 75 g **c.** 10 g
- **(4) a.** 100 g **b.** 75 **c.** 84 g
- **(5)** 15 g
- **(6) a.** 100 ml **b.** 125 ml
- **(7) a.** 5% **b.** 1·5% **c.** 0·2%
- **(8)** 80 ml
- **(9)** 15 ml

Chapter 5: Drip rates

EXERCISE 5A
- **(1)** 20 drops/min   **(2)** 50 drops/min
- **(3)** 50 drops/min   **(4)** 4 hours
- **(5)** 5 hours   **(6)** $8\frac{1}{3}$ hours = 8 h 20 min

EXERCISE 5B   All answers in drops/min.
- **(1)** 50   **(2)** 25   **(3)** $62\frac{1}{2} \Rightarrow 63$
- **(4)** $37\frac{1}{2} \Rightarrow 38$ **(5)** $43\frac{3}{4} \Rightarrow 44$

EXERCISE 5C   All answers in drops/min
- **(1)** 25   **(2)** $18\frac{3}{4} \Rightarrow 19$ **(3)** $31\frac{1}{4} \Rightarrow 32$
- **(4)** $37\frac{1}{2} \Rightarrow 38$ **(5)** $16\frac{2}{3} \Rightarrow 17$ **(6)** $28\frac{1}{8} \Rightarrow 29$
- **(7)** $18\frac{3}{4} \Rightarrow 19$ **(8)** 15   **(9)** $9\frac{3}{8} \Rightarrow 10$
- **(10)** $15\frac{5}{8} \Rightarrow 16$ **(11)** $31\frac{1}{4} \Rightarrow 32$ **(12)** 35
- **(13)** $41\frac{1}{3} \Rightarrow 42$ **(14)** $20\frac{5}{6} \Rightarrow 21$

EXERCISE 5D
- **(1)** 1800ml   **(2)** 1872 ml
- **(3)** $6 h + 8\frac{1}{2} h = 14\frac{1}{2}$ h   **(4)** 10 h + 5 h = 15 h
- **(5)** Runs 13 h; finishes 2100 hours   **(6)** Runs $14\frac{1}{2}$ h; finishes 1830 hours
- **(7)** $37\frac{1}{2}$ drops/min $\Rightarrow$ 38 drops/min   **(8)** $16\frac{1}{4}$ drops/min $\Rightarrow$ 17 drops/min

Chapter 6: Paediatric dosages

EXERCISE 6A   All answers in milligrams
  (1) 120   **(2)** 150   **(3)** 90
  (4) 250   **(5)** 300   **(6)** 400
  (7) 900   **(8)** 480   **(9)** 540

EXERCISE 6B   All answers in millilitres
  (1) 0·4   **(2)** 0·4   **(3)** 0·8   **(4)** 0·75
  (5) 0·5   **(6)** 0·72   **(7)** 0·4   **(8)** 0·75
  (9) 0·48   **(10)** 1·2   **(11)** 1·2   **(12)** 0·3
(13) 0·25   **(14)** 0·6   **(15)** 0·65 **(16)** 1·5
(17) 1·0   **(18)** 0·8   **(19)** 0·6   **(20)** 0·8

EXERCISE 6C   All answers in millilitres
  (1) 3·5   **(2)** 12·5   **(3)** 6   **(4)** 9
  (5) 2·5   **(6)** 8   **(7)** 14   **(8)** 3
  (9) 4   **(10)** $6\frac{2}{3}$ or 6·7

Chapter 7: Summary exercises

SUMMARY EXERCISE 1

  (1) 4.5 ml   **(2)** 0.5 ml
  (3) $1\frac{1}{2}$ tablets   **(4)** 14 ml
  (5) $\frac{1}{8}$ or 1 in 8   **(6)** **a.** 250 ml **b.** 4750 ml
  (7) **a.** 500 ml **b.** 2000 ml **(8)** **a.** 150 ml **b.** 1050 ml
  (9) 50g   **(10)** $21\frac{7}{8}$ ⇒ 22 drops/min
(11) 5 h + $7\frac{1}{2}$ h = $12\frac{1}{2}$ h **(12)** 225mg/dose
(13) 0.7 ml   **(14)** 0.35 ml
(15) 2.5 ml

SUMMARY EXERCISE 2

  (1) 0·9 ml   **(2)** $\frac{1}{2}$ tablet
  (3) 18 ml   **(4)** 0.5%
  (5) 4%   **(6)** **a.** 1·6 ml **b.** 2·4 ml
  (7) **a.** 20 ml **b.** 780 ml **(8)** 120 ml Savlon; 2280 ml water
  (9) 1750 ml   **(10)** $6\frac{1}{4}$ hours
(11) 12 h + 5 h = 17 h   **(12)** 320mg/dose
(13) 1·4 ml   **(14)** 6 ml
(15) 7 ml

Short list of mathematical terms

Whole numbers

WHOLE NUMBER
> A number without fractions, e.g. 5, 17, 438, 10 592.
> Whole numbers are also known as *integers*.

Vulgar fractions

VULGAR FRACTION
> Also known as a common fraction.
> e.g. $\frac{3}{8}$, $\frac{17}{5}$, $\frac{1}{6}$, $\frac{9}{4000}$

NUMERATOR
> The top number in a vulgar fraction.
> e.g. In the fraction $\frac{3}{8}$ the numerator is 3.

DENOMINATOR
> The bottom number in a vulgar fraction.
> e.g. In the fraction $\frac{3}{8}$ the denominator is 8.

MIXED NUMBER
> Partly a whole number, partly a fraction.
> e.g. $1\frac{5}{8}$, $4\frac{1}{2}$, $10\frac{17}{50}$

Decimals

DECIMAL
> Generally used to mean a number which includes a decimal point.
> e.g. 6·35, 0·748, 0·002, 236·5

DECIMAL PLACES
> Numbers to the right of the decimal point.
> e.g. 6·35 has 2 decimal places
> > 0·748 has 3 decimal places
> > 0·002 has 3 decimal places
> > 236·5 has one decimal place

PLACE VALUE (IN DECIMALS)
> To the right of the decimal point are tenths, hundredths, thousandths, etc....
> e.g. In the number 0·962, there are 9 tenths, 6 hundredths and 2 thousandths.

Percentages

PERCENTAGE

Number of parts per hundred parts.

e.g. 14% means 14 parts per 100 parts

2·5% means 2·5 parts per 100 parts

A percentage may be less than 1%

e.g. 0·3% means 0·3 parts per 100 = 3 parts per 1000

0·04% means 0·04 parts per 100 = 4 parts per 10 000.

Other terms

DIVISOR

The number by which you are dividing.

e.g. In the division 495 ÷ 15, the divisor is 15.

EVALUATE

Calculate; find the value. The answer will be a number.

SIMPLIFY

Write as simply as possible.

Commonly used SI (metric) prefixes

PREFIX	SYMBOL	FACTOR	EXAMPLE
mega	M	1 000 000	2·5 megaunits (Mu) = 2 500 000 units
kilo	K	1000	3 kilograms (Kg) = 3000 grams
milli	m	0.001 (thousandth)	5 millilitre (ml) = $0·005 = \frac{5}{1000}$ litre
micro	μ*	0·000 001 (millionth)	40 micrograms = $0·000\ 04 = \frac{40}{1000\ 000}$ gram

* Always write 'micro' in full. Using 'μ' can cause errors.